100 Questions & Answers About Your Child's Epilepsy

Anuradha Singh, MD

NYU Comprehensive Epilepsy Center
New York, NY

JONES AND BARTLETT PUBLISHERS
Sudbury, Massachusetts
BOSTON   TORONTO   LONDON   SINGAPORE

World Headquarters

Jones and Bartlett Publishers	Jones and Bartlett Publishers	Jones and Bartlett Publishers
40 Tall Pine Drive	Canada	International
Sudbury, MA 01776	6339 Ormindale Way	Barb House, Barb Mews
978-443-5000	Mississauga, Ontario L5V 1J2	London W6 7PA
info@jbpub.com	Canada	United Kingdom
www.jbpub.com		

Jones and Bartlett's books and products are available through most bookstores and online booksellers. To contact Jones and Bartlett Publishers directly, call 800-832-0034, fax 978-443-8000, or visit our website, www.jbpub.com.

Substantial discounts on bulk quantities of Jones and Bartlett's publications are available to corporations, professional associations, and other qualified organizations. For details and specific discount information, contact the special sales department at Jones and Bartlett via the above contact information or send an email to specialsales@jbpub.com.

The authors, editor, and publisher have made every effort to provide accurate information. However, they are not responsible for errors, omissions, or for any outcomes related to the use of the contents of this book and take no responsibility for the use of the products and procedures described. Treatments and side effects described in this book may not be applicable to all people; likewise, some people may require a dose or experience a side effect that is not described herein. Drugs and medical devices are discussed that may have limited availability controlled by the Food and Drug Administration (FDA) for use only in a research study or clinical trial. Research, clinical practice, and government regulations often change the accepted standard in this field. When consideration is being given to use of any drug in the clinical setting, the healthcare provider or reader is responsible for determining FDA status of the drug, reading the package insert, and reviewing prescribing information for the most up-to-date recommendations on dose, precautions, and contraindications, and determining the appropriate usage for the product. This is especially important in the case of drugs that are new or seldom used.

Production Credits
Executive Publisher: Christopher Davis
Senior Editorial Assistant: Jessica Acox
Production Editor: Daniel Stone
Manufacturing and Inventory Control Supervisor: Amy Bacus
Composition: Maggie Dana/Pageworks
Printing: Malloy, Inc.
Cover Printing: Malloy, Inc.

Cover Credits
Cover Design: Carolyn Downer
Top Photo: © Ersler Dmitry/ShutterStock, Inc.; Bottom Left Photo: © Courtnee Mulroy/ShutterStock, Inc.; and Bottom Right Photo: LiquidLibrary

Library of Congress Cataloging-in-Publication Data
Singh, Anuradha.
   100 questions and answers about your child's epilepsy / Anuradha Singh.
       p. cm.
   Includes bibliographical references and index.
   ISBN-13: 978-0-7637-5521-8
   ISBN-10: 0-7637-5521-4
   1. Epilepsy in children—Miscellanea. 2. Epileptic children—Miscellanea. I. Title.
II. Title: One hundred questions and answers about your child's epilepsy.
   RJ496.E6S56   2009
   618.92'853—dc22

                                                          2008028672

6048

Printed in the United States of America
12 11 10 09 08 10 9 8 7 6 5 4 3 2 1

CONTENTS

Growing Up with Epilepsy: A Patient's Story

Epilepsy and seizures have been a major part of most of my life. I am now a 36-year-old man who has been seizure free for nearly 4 years, and I have had complex partial seizures since around the age of 6–8 years old—probably earlier than that, but 6–8 is about as far back as I can remember them.

At that time nobody knew something was unusual except for me. My seizures were short and typically characterized by a strange rising sensation in my stomach, staring off into space for anywhere from 30 seconds to a few minutes, and various degrees of disorientation afterward. By the time somebody noticed that I was "spacing out" I was often coming out of my seizure and could jump right back into a conversation (although perhaps with some awkwardness since I might not recall what had just been said).

I can remember playing kickball around the age of 10 years old. At that time I was undiagnosed. I recall the rising sensation, while standing on first base, then everybody screaming for me to run. Feeling extremely confused, I began to run home and didn't stop until I was almost there.

At a doctor's appointment later that year, I brought it up. I described the funny feeling I got in my stomach. I had little idea that I was staring into space or about any other symptoms. My doctor suggested bismuth (Pepto-Bismol) to help with my stomach.

Looking back, I am sure that some friends knew something was up but at that age nobody knew what to do or say.

For years after that, I continued to have seizures, undiagnosed until one day I was playing a video game in front of my father. It was a racing game, and I pulled the vehicle over to the side of the track. My dad watched and asked me several times what I was doing (I don't recall this). After about a minute, I snapped out of it, finished the race (in last place) and ambled out of the arcade as if nothing unusual had happened. My father looked at me puzzled and asked what had just happened. I wasn't quite sure what he meant. After he recapped what he had seen, I remembered, and I exclaimed, "That was the funny feeling I have been telling you about all of these years!"

Finally the dots were connected and at the age of 14 there was a diagnosis. The medication I was prescribed controlled my seizures (except when, as a forgetful and rebellious teenager, I would not take my meds).

Later in my teens, my seizures came back and epilepsy became much more ingrained in my identity. Although sometimes embarrassed by it, I did my best to keep a joking façade to my friends and not make it such a big deal. For the most part they played along. Still, even among my knowing friends, drooling into my dinner plate for 2 minutes was never something I felt good about, even if I made light of it afterward and got a laugh.

I did finally get serious about my health and began keeping a detailed account of every episode. Armed with detailed data, my doctors and I tried new medication combinations. I was referred to a comprehensive epilepsy center, and finally, years later . . . brain surgery, which was both extremely challenging and extremely rewarding.

As a medical exercise, it was a huge success. I have had only two seizures since the operation 4 years ago (as compared to 3–5 a week prior to surgery). The procedure and the recovery itself, though, were physically and emotionally challenging.

The gifts I could not have predicted are the many people who have approached me since my surgery. Having navigated through that event, and through the arc of my experience as a whole, I have been placed in a somewhat unique position to help others. I have been privileged to meet several people who have undergone similar procedures since mine and to share my own experiences with them.

Jared Caponi

Epilepsy: A Child–Parent Perspective
A Young Patient's Perspective

My name is Packy Jones. I am 14 years old and have been a patient of Dr. Singh since I was 11.

When I was first diagnosed with epilepsy 4 years ago, I had many fears, questions, etc. My first thought was, "Why me?" Well, I know now that that question will never be answered, but many others have been. Plus, I have also realized that I can get through this—my seizures—because it could be so much worse. I have had ten grand mal, tonic-clonic seizures since November 2004. Some people have ten seizures a day, so I try to consider myself one of the lucky ones.

The day I was officially diagnosed with epilepsy presenting with tonic-clonic seizures was one I will never forget. I had so many fears for my future, but only three major ones. My biggest fear was that I would no longer be able to play hockey. There is no seizure history in my family; I had no tumor and no injuries to my head. We had no idea why I seized. I was really worried that the doctors would not let me play because we didn't know when I was going to seize, and they wanted me to be safe. As it turned out, however, I was able to play. After missing an entire season (five months), the doctors cleared me to play, and I was ready to hit the ice. I had to be more cautious the first few months, but that was okay by me. I eventually played just like I always had, and I continue to play all the time.

My second major fear was that my bedtime curfew would always be so early. In the beginning, I had to be in bed asleep by 7:30 p.m., and I worried that would be true my entire life. I did (and do) know that a seizure trigger is lack of sleep, but we didn't know what was triggering mine. What if it wasn't little sleep? Either way, though, it was better to be safe and take it slow until everyone was sure I could stay up later. All the doctors said that the longer I went seizure free, the later I would be able to stay up. So, I was determined to follow all the rules so that my bedtime could approach normal. Gradually it was moved to 8:00 p.m., then 8:30 p.m., then 9:00 p.m. After 2 years without a seizure, I am now able to stay up a bit later, so long as I am in bed asleep by 10 p.m. I know that most people—especially teenagers—think this is early, but, for me, I am thrilled and grateful.

My third major fear was the way I would be treated by the people around me. Would I be treated differently now? Poorly? Normally? Would people think I was strange, a freak even? I wasn't sure. One thing that I was sure about, though, was that I really wanted to be treated the way I always had. My parents, brothers, and sister tried to assure me that nothing would change, but I found it hard to believe. All the stories about what I looked like and what I did during my seizures went through my mind. I *was* treated differently in the beginning, but not in a bad way—I just had to be closely watched. In time, though, my friends, teachers, and other family members all treated me the same way they always had. Other than a few occasional questions, everything is back to how it was before my first seizure, and that is just fine by me!

All in all, the beginning of a seizure disorder is the hardest— *definitely* the hardest—part, because there are so many unanswered questions and fears. As time goes on, you get used to the rules, guidelines, terms, and everything else about them. You realize (I know I did!) that as long as you do what the doctors suggest, have your parents help you, and talk with people about your situation, it's not all that bad. It could always be worse, and laughing is what gets me through.

Packy Jones, age 14

A Mother's Story

November 4th, 2004, changed the life of our family forever. The phone rang a little after 8 a.m. It was the middle school nurse asking me to come to the school—Packy (our 11-year-old son and oldest of our five children) had a 3-minute-long seizure. In a panic and flurry we went to him. We got a friend to watch our four younger children, and we sped to the school. Over the next few hours and days, I tried to calm my fears. I thought, "It wasn't a seizure." "He fainted." "His electrolytes were too low." "He hit his head and passed out." Anything but a seizure. I am not sure why that word was so scary to me then, but it was. All sorts of questions about his future went through my mind, too. If it was a seizure, I wondered, "What does this mean for Packy?" "For our other four children?" "For our family?" "For his schooling?" "His hockey?" "His preteen life?" "What about the future?" "Will he drive?" "How can I fix this? . . . *How can I fix this?*"

Packy had an EEG, MRI, and neuro testing within days. Within the week, the diagnosis came: "Packy, your MRI is normal." *Oh, thank God!* "But, you did have a seizure. You have a tonic-clonic seizure disorder."

My stomach sank. Packy's face fell. My husband, Michael, sat motionless in his chair. Packy only had one question: "Can I still play hockey?"

"Not for a while, Packy," the doctor answered. "We need to get medicine in you first."

My heart never felt so sad. I was so angry, irate. I wanted to rip that doctor's face off—like somehow it was his fault. I realized quickly that that wouldn't solve anything, so I went right to work. Researching everything about tonic-clonic seizures, medicines, protocols, research, dos and don'ts—everything. We were determined to have Packy be, and grow up, as normal as any other 11-year-old. We came up with systems for everything. He wasn't allowed to be alone—anywhere—ever. So we devised a routine for the bathroom; we had one of his friends stop by the house every morning to walk with him to school; and Michael got back on the ice to coach so Packy could at least skate at his practices (all this with the doctor's approval, of course). After Packy's third seizure—they were coming more frequently now—I called the NYU Comprehensive Epilepsy Center. Packy's neurologist at home just wasn't helping the way I knew someone could. We met Dr. Singh and found instant peace and comfort. They assured us—him, really—that letting him be an 11-year-old boy was the best way to treat him.

We have worked hard over the past 4 years to do that—all with Dr. Singh's help. I still worry, though. I have come to realize that that won't go away. I worry he will seize. I worry he's on too much medicine. I worry he won't drive. I worry he won't reach his dream of playing college hockey. I worry about my other children. I guess I worry a lot, but I don't let it consume me. We go through the emotions of what we have to do and when it comes to normal teenage stuff, we explore other safe options for him. But, mostly, we just let Packy be Packy.

It's been an interesting path so far, and I assume it will continue to be. We learned that we need to find humor in this often and laugh every day. We continue to find safe ways in this, and we stay up on all information on his seizures, treatments, and epilepsy. I know my son will grow to be an incredible man. He's already on his way. I wish it would be an easy, care-free path for him, but it's not and that's become okay with us. We take comfort by believing there must be a reason for this. Some of his hopes and dreams have had to shift since November of 2004, but that's life. It makes me sad sometimes, but I don't let him know that. We focus on the *cans*, not the cannots. It helps make it easier. As of today, Packy has had ten grand mal tonic-clonic seizures. We hope that ten will be his number—that he won't have any more. We are regimented about his sleep and his meds—the only two things that we *can* control. The rest of it, we take as it comes, trying to find a way to laugh along the way. It doesn't make sense for us to worry about bad things. Every day we make a decision to focus on the good and it's getting us through . . . getting us through.

Lynne Jones, *Packy's mother*

About 2–2.3 million people in the United States suffer from epilepsy; one-third of them are children. What do seizures mean to children and to their parents? During my fellowship training years, I was touched by something that I want to share with my readers. A child had been admitted to the epilepsy unit for management of infantile spasms. The child had very subtle spasms, which made it difficult for nurses and doctors to recognize on the video clips. During the course of her night, the child's mother tried to sleep next to her daughter. It was a very moving experience in that the mother was so attentive to fluctuations in her daughter's condition, that she didn't allow herself to rest. Whenever her daughter had a brief seizure—one that lasted hardly 2 seconds— she jumped up and called for immediate help. Throughout the night she was jotting down what she saw and the time each seizure occurred in a seizure log book. Every time the mother called for help, she had correctly recognized and identified a seizure. Her daughter had a brief spasm that showed as a seizure on the EEG. Because these are sometimes very brief, they are difficult to recognize on a video. By the end of the night, the mother had pushed the seizure alarm 30–50 times.

It is hard to imagine parents of children with epilepsy going through this night after night. It is a parent's nightmare to watch his or her child having a seizure, turning blue, or biting his or her tongue. Those at the extremes of age—the elderly and children— are the most vulnerable to having seizures. Quality of life issues are closely intertwined with the frequency, severity, and chronicity of seizures. There is an overwhelming need to provide patients and their caregivers with more information about and a better understanding of epilepsy. It is increasingly recognized that the burden of seizures is based upon the perception of seizure control rather than actual seizure control.

Physicians may be hard pressed for time to discuss the full impact seizures have on a child's health and development. During short office visits, the physician may or may not fulfill the emotional needs of the children who do not understand what their illness is, of adolescents who see their dreams shattered by new diagnoses, or of overprotective parents who start blaming themselves for their child's epilepsy. Teachers and school professionals are often unaware of and not equipped to handle seizures at school.

In this book, I have tried to provide patients, families, and caregivers with up-to-date information about basic understanding of mechanisms of epilepsy. Seizure types, diagnostic tests, and treatment modalities are discussed in detail. About 20–30% of patients are refractory to medications. Early surgical intervention is the key to help some of these children with intractable epilepsy.

ACKNOWLEDGMENTS

I sincerely thank my patients and their families who inspired me to write this book. Packy Jones, Lynne Jones, and Jared Caponi deserve special acknowledgment for their valuable commentary in the book.

I am also indebted to William MacAllister, PhD, Neuropsychologist, and Howard Weiner MD, Associate Professor of Neurosurgery and Pediatrics, at NYU Medical Center for their valuable contributions to my book.

Anuradha Singh

PART ONE

Basics of Epilepsy

I am not sure if my child has epilepsy or not. What is the difference between seizures and epilepsy?

My family has no history of seizures. How did my daughter develop this problem? What could be the cause of her seizures?

What else can it be, if what seems to be seizures actually aren't?

More ...

1. I am not sure if my child has epilepsy or not. What is the difference between seizures and epilepsy?

A **seizure** is defined as any change in clinical behavior as a result of hyperexcitation of the brain cells. This abnormal clinical behavior may vary from something very subtle to a more obvious strong seizure such as a **grand mal seizure**. The patient usually returns to his or her normal state after a brief period of altered responsiveness after the seizure is over. This stage is called the **postictal state** (from post, meaning after, and **ictus**, meaning seizure). The duration of the postictal state can really vary from patient to patient and may last from a couple of seconds to hours. Some patients describe how they do not feel like themselves for a few days after the seizures.

Seizures originate in the brain. The brain and spinal cord are part of the **central nervous system**. The brain has **cerebral hemispheres** (right and left) and a lower part called the **brain stem** (**Figure 1**). The hemispheres have an outer surface called **cortex** or **gray matter**. The cortex is made of neuron cells. It is believed that there are 100 billion **neurons** in the human brain. These neurons are connected very intricately to each other, thus allowing the neurons to communicate with each other. The inner part of the cerebral hemispheres is composed of **white matter** and fluid-filled spaces called **ventricles**. Seizures originate in the cortex, but white matter plays a crucial role in the propagation of seizures. The communication between the neurons is polarized and occurs at the contact points, which are called **synapses**. The neurons release chemicals called **neurotransmitters** around these synapses. Neurotransmitters can cause excitation or inhibition. The firing neurons can cause

seizure

An abnormal clinical behavior as a result of excessive excitation of brain cells.

grand mal seizure

A sudden attack or convulsion characterized by generalized muscle spasms and loss of consciousness.

postictal state

A state immediately after seizure is over.

ictus

A sudden event, such as a seizure, collapse, or faint.

central nervous system

The portion of the vertebrate nervous system consisting of the brain and spinal cord.

cerebral hemispheres

Two parts of the brain (right and left).

brain stem

Lower part of the brain.

cortex

The outer layer of gray matter that covers the surface of the cerebral hemisphere.

gray matter

The outer surface of the cerebral hemisphere composed of cell bodies of neurons.

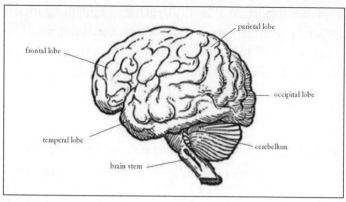

Figure 1
Cerebral hemispheres and brain stem.

excitatory or inhibitory electrical impulses. The sums of excitatory and inhibitory impulses determine the state of brain cells. Seizures result when the excitation overpowers inhibition. Seizures occur when there is sudden, ~~~~~~~~~~~~~~ of discharges of gray matter.

~~~~~~~~~~~ udden change in ~~~~~~~~~ ensation—a sud- ~~~~~~~~ s reversible and ~~~~~~~~ nutes. The impli- ~~~~~~~~~ rent for provoked

~~~~~~~~ provoked, **parox-** ~~~~~ the same question ~~~~~~~ out the difference ~~~~~~ f social stigmata is ~~~~~~ ilepsy is like many ~~~~~ h as **diabetes mel-** ~~~~~ outgrow epilepsy.

~~~~~~~~~~~ ple in the United
States an~~~~~~~~~~~~~~~~~~~~~~~~~~~~~~ ty children. It is a

neuron

Building block of the brain made up of a cell body, the axon, and the dendrites.

white matter

One of the three components of the brain.

ventricles

Hollow cavities in the brain filled with cerebrospinal fluid.

synapses

Contact points where the communication between neurons is polarized.

neurotransmitter

Small-molecular-weight compound that conveys messages across a synapse.

epilepsy

A neurological condition in which a person has a tendency to have repeated seizures—more than two that are unprovoked.

paroxysmal

Characterized by a sudden outburst or eruption.

diabetes mellitus

Diabetes caused by a relative or absolute deficiency of insulin (a hormone secreted by the pancreas).

treatable condition. Most (70–80%) of epilepsy patients are well controlled on just one or two antiepileptics. The other 20–30% may not find adequate medical therapy and require diagnostic testing to confirm the diagnosis and determine the treatment strategies.

2. My family has no history of seizures. How did my daughter develop this problem? What could be the cause of her seizures?

Your daughter can have epilepsy even if there was no other family member affected by epilepsy. Some cases of epilepsy are inherited, and some are not. Seizures can occur at any age. However, the vulnerability to seizures may vary by age. There are different stages in a child's development, which include the following:

Fetus (after the second month of pregnancy)
Neonate (first 28 days of life after birth)
Infant (after 28 days of life until 1 year of age)
Toddler (1 to 2 years of age)
Preschool years (2 years to 6 years of age)
School years (6 years to 18 years of age)

Causes of epilepsy differ with different stages of development. **Childhood epilepsy syndromes** are recognized by the age of onset, seizure types, and their EEG pattern.

All epilepsies do not have to be familial or genetically predetermined. There could be several causes for seizures in children as listed in **Table 1**. Your daughter may be predisposed to seizures because of the birth trauma during delivery. Hypoxia or lack of oxygen can cause brain injuries. Inborn metabolic disorders of pro-

childhood epilepsy syndromes

These are age-related syndromes that tend to have a clinical onset at a certain age, particular seizure type (s), and a unique EEG pattern. It is important to recognize these syndromes to be able to understand the best treatment options and their prognosis.

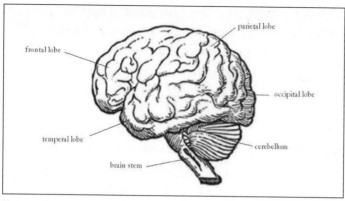

Figure 1
Cerebral hemispheres and brain stem.

excitatory or inhibitory electrical impulses. The sums of excitatory and inhibitory impulses determine the state of brain cells. Seizures result when the excitation overpowers inhibition. Seizures occur when there is sudden, excessive synchronization of discharges of gray matter. Clinically, a seizure can manifest as a sudden change in behavior, emotion, motor function, or sensation—a sudden change from the baseline that is reversible and unprovoked and lasts for seconds to minutes. The implications and treatment options are different for provoked and unprovoked seizures.

Epilepsy is defined as two or more unprovoked, **paroxysmal** seizures. A lot of patients ask the same question you have asked and are not clear about the difference between seizures and epilepsy. A lot of social stigmata is attached to the term *epilepsy*. But epilepsy is like many other chronic medical conditions such as **diabetes mellitus** or hypertension. Some children outgrow epilepsy.

Epilepsy affects 2 to 4 million people in the United States and affects about one in fifty children. It is a

neuron
Building block of the brain made up of a cell body, the axon, and the dendrites.

white matter
One of the three components of the brain.

ventricles
Hollow cavities in the brain filled with cerebrospinal fluid.

synapses
Contact points where the communication between neurons is polarized.

neurotransmitter
Small-molecular-weight compound that conveys messages across a synapse.

epilepsy
A neurological condition in which a person has a tendency to have repeated seizures—more than two that are unprovoked.

paroxysmal
Characterized by a sudden outburst or eruption.

diabetes mellitus
Diabetes caused by a relative or absolute deficiency of insulin (a hormone secreted by the pancreas).

Basics of Epilepsy

treatable condition. Most (70–80%) of epilepsy patients are well controlled on just one or two antiepileptics. The other 20–30% may not find adequate medical therapy and require diagnostic testing to confirm the diagnosis and determine the treatment strategies.

2. My family has no history of seizures. How did my daughter develop this problem? What could be the cause of her seizures?

Your daughter can have epilepsy even if there was no other family member affected by epilepsy. Some cases of epilepsy are inherited, and some are not. Seizures can occur at any age. However, the vulnerability to seizures may vary by age. There are different stages in a child's development, which include the following:

Fetus (after the second month of pregnancy)
Neonate (first 28 days of life after birth)
Infant (after 28 days of life until 1 year of age)
Toddler (1 to 2 years of age)
Preschool years (2 years to 6 years of age)
School years (6 years to 18 years of age)

Causes of epilepsy differ with different stages of development. **Childhood epilepsy syndromes** are recognized by the age of onset, seizure types, and their EEG pattern.

childhood epilepsy syndromes

These are age-related syndromes that tend to have a clinical onset at a certain age, particular seizure type (s), and a unique EEG pattern. It is important to recognize these syndromes to be able to understand the best treatment options and their prognosis.

All epilepsies do not have to be familial or genetically predetermined. There could be several causes for seizures in children as listed in **Table 1**. Your daughter may be predisposed to seizures because of the birth trauma during delivery. Hypoxia or lack of oxygen can cause brain injuries. Inborn metabolic disorders of pro-

Basics of Epilepsy

Table 1   Causes of Epileptic Seizures
• Congenital
• Degenerative
• Genetic
• Idiopathic
• Infections
• Metabolic
• Injuries during childbirth
• Tumors
• Trauma
• Toxic
• Vascular (like stroke before or after birth, blood vessel abnormalities)

teins, carbohydrates, fats causing neurological dysfunction, and seizures could be another possibility. Some patients develop seizures early on with high fever. These are called **febrile seizures**. Other children may have seizures associated with developmental delays or learning disabilities. Seizures may develop after severe head trauma with loss of consciousness. This condition is called **posttraumatic epilepsy**. Seizures may happen soon after the head trauma or can occur after a latent period of months to years. The risk of head trauma is higher if the patient has loss of consciousness or has no memory of the head trauma. Head trauma can be mild, moderate, or severe.

Mild: brief period of unconsciousness or loss of memory.

Moderate: 30 minutes to 24 hours of loss of consciousness or loss of memory; skull fracture.

Severe: bruising of the brain, bleeding in the brain or coverings of the brain; more than 24 hours of loss of consciousness or loss of memory.

Significant head trauma causing bleeding in the brain or around the brain coverings increases the chances of developing posttraumatic epilepsy. Bleeding in the brain

febrile seizures
Seizures in association with high fever.

posttraumatic epilepsy
Seizures resulting from head trauma.

meninges

Three coverings of the brain.

meningitis

Inflammation of the meninges.

encephalitis

Inflammation of the brain tissue.

focal seizure

Seizure coming from one discrete focus or part of the brain.

brain tumors

Abnormal proliferation of brain cells, neurons, or supporting cells (glia).

partial seizures

Seizures in which the abnormal electrical activity begins in one part of the brain.

tonic-clonic seizures

Generalized seizures; also called convulsion or grand mal.

hypothalamus

Part of the brain that controls many bodily functions such as temperature, sleep, sexual functions, and food intake.

pituitary gland

The master gland of the endocrine system. It is located at the base of the brain.

can leave behind an area of scar tissue or a cavity that can cause epilepsy at a later age.

Children may acquire infections of the brain. Infection of the brain coverings (called **meninges**) is called **meningitis**. Infection or inflammation of the brain is called **encephalitis** (encephalon means brain). Sometimes, there is clear-cut pathology in the brain explaining predisposition to seizures. For example, images of the brain can detect benign or malignant tumors, old scar tissue, or signs of brain injury or abnormal blood vessels in the brain. Tumors are a rare cause of seizures in children, and they do not account for more than 5% of **focal seizures**. Children who have **brain tumors** tend to have them in the lower part of the brain called brain stem. About 10–15% of children with brain tumors can present with a **partial seizure** or a **tonic-clonic seizure**. Tumors arising from the **hypothalamus** (the part of the brain that controls our master gland or **pituitary gland**) are associated with **gelastic seizures** (sudden laughter or display of strong emotions). Tumors can present with partial **status epilepticus** (nonstop seizures from part of the brain that do not stop on their own) that is known as **epilepsia partialis continua. Strokes** in the brain may develop while the fetus is developing in the uterus or may occur later on in life. As the brain develops, there has to be proper migration and arrangement of cells in the brain called neurons. Too little or too much at a certain place in the brain can cause what we call **neuronal migrational disorders.** These can be focal or more diffuse and are detected by neuroimaging. When the cause of seizures can be localized, it is called **localization-related epilepsy**. Sometimes we suspect a cause for epilepsy but cannot determine it by the diagnostic tools available to us, no matter how hard we look. This is called cryptic (meaning indeterminate). It is hard to predict who will develop epilepsy in the future.

Epilepsy is a very common condition; about 50 new cases are seen per 100,000 people per year. In the United States, epilepsy consumes 12.5 billion dollars per year. This includes both direct and indirect costs.

3. What else can it be, if what seems to be seizures actually aren't?

Not everything that shakes is a seizure. Seizures remain undiagnosed for longer than 6 months for about 50% of the patients with epilepsy. Very young children do some strange repetitive behaviors that can be confused with seizures. **Table 2** lists several disorders that emulate

Table 2   Recurrent Episodes That Imitate Epilepsy
• Jitteriness (in the newborn period)
• Gastroesophageal reflux (Sandifer's syndrome)
• Breath-holding spasms/apneic attacks
• Nonepileptic seizures (psychogenic seizures)
• Transient ischemic attacks
• Hypoglycemia (low glucose)
• Movement disorders: tics, chorea, dystonia, periodic leg movements, restless leg syndrome
• Sleep disorders—sleep walking, nightmares, night terrors, benign sleep myoclonus
• Shuddering attacks
• Rigors (with fever)
• Head banging
• Startle responses
• Bruxism
• Panic attacks, anxiety, or rage attacks
• Delirium
• Cardiac arrhythmias
• Migraine
• Syncope
• Drop attacks
• Narcolepsy/cataplexy
• Self-stimulatory behavior—masturbation, mannerisms, rhythmic motor habits

Basics of Epilepsy

gelastic seizures

Seizures with brief outbursts of emotions, either laughing or crying without any mirth.

status epilepticus

Seizures continuing for a prolonged time, usually more than 30 minutes, without returning to baseline.

epilepsia partialis continua

Continuous seizure activity originating from one side of the brain. Patients may be completely aware of their surroundings. This condition is commonly seen in patients with brain tumors.

stroke

Death of brain tissue that usually results from obstruction to the blood flow of the brain.

neuronal migrational disorder

Any defect in the development or the migration or the laying down of the brain cells called neurons.

localization-related epilepsy

Focal or partial seizure.

vasovagal attack

A temporary vascular reaction associated with rapid fall in heart rate and blood pressure.

benign neonatal sleep myoclonus

A self-limiting disorder in neonates characterized by myoclonic jerks.

benign sleep myoclonus

A distinctive disorder of sleep in infancy characterized by rhythmic myoclonic jerks (sudden muscle contractions) that occur when the child is asleep and stop when the child is awakened.

dystonia

Abnormal tone of muscle.

periodic leg movements

Repetitive leg movements of sleep, almost occurring every 20 to 40 seconds which can last a few minutes to several hours.

restless leg syndrome

Unpleasant sensation in the legs that occurs when retiring to bed.

bruxism

Teeth grinding at night.

epilepsy. These can occur during daytime or at night, whether the child is awake or asleep. **Vasovagal attack** is a common cause of loss of consciousness in young children precipitated by extreme physical or emotional stressors, fear, anxiety, pain, etc.

Children may have repeated episodes of head banging. Typically head banging appears in the latter half of the first year of life. These movements are common in children with developmental disorders or in autistic children. Head banging is more common in males and generally ends by preschool age. Stereotyped movements such as head rolling and body rocking are common during infancy. Infants may display a very common phenomenon called jitteriness of the whole body, especially if the mother had a history of drug abuse or was on any antiepileptics. Brief, rapid jerks called **benign neonatal myoclonus** can be confused with seizures. **Benign sleep myoclonus** (sleep jerks) during infancy can be mistaken for seizures. Movements can involve both sides, can spread from one body part to the other, and may have involvement of big as well as small muscles.

There is another gamut of disorders that are grouped under movement disorders. Different body parts can exhibit abnormal posturing, which is termed **dystonia**. These movements completely disappear as soon as the child wakes up from sleep. **Periodic leg movements** and **restless leg syndrome** can be seen in older children during light stages of sleep. Grinding of teeth, called **bruxism**, can be misdiagnosed for seizurelike activity. **Masturbation** is another self-stimulation behavior that is commonly confused with epilepsy or movement disorders. It is common in infants and young children. Very young infants may get pleasure in stimulating genitals just like thumb-sucking behavior. The peak age of masturbation is at age 4 years and again during adolescence. It is believed that 80–90% of males and 40–50% of females have masturbated at some point in life. Children may perform rhythmic stereotyped movements, which could be very subtle and confusing. Brief staring into space, body stiffening, thrusting hip movements on the floor, mild grunting, and abnormal posturing of arms, neck, and legs can raise suspicion of seizures. These behaviors may cease when children are distracted or engaged in other activities.

Disorders of respiration such as episodes of **apnea** are common in infants and children. Apnea is cessation of breathing. A child who stops breathing might turn blue. Obstruction in the airway can cause apnea. Breathing is also controlled by respiratory centers in the lower part of the brain. Periods of apnea without any changes on the **electroencephalogram (EEG)** are not epileptic in nature.

Sleep walking, **sleep talking**, nightmares, and **night terrors** in children can be confused with abnormal behavior seen during seizures. **Narcolepsy**, a disorder of sleep, can present during adolescence and has to be differentiated from epilepsy. Narcolepsy has four components, which are:

1. Excessive daytime sleepiness
2. **Cataplexy**: transient decrease in muscle tone without loss of consciousness
3. Vivid dreams
4. Sleep paralysis: inability to move during transition from wakefulness to sleep and vice versa

---

masturbation
Sexual self-gratification; manipulation of one's own genitals manually or by other means to achieve orgasm.

apnea
Cessation of breathing.

electroencephalogram (EEG)
Graphic representation of brain waves revealing the functional status of the brain.

sleep walking
Walking while asleep or in a sleeplike state; also called somnambulism.

sleep talking
Uttering speech while sleep. This is also called "somniloquy."

night terrors
Episodes of extreme fear, anxiety, or panic within a few hours after going to sleep.

narcolepsy
Excessive daytime sleepiness and disturbed nighttime sleep.

cataplexy
A sudden loss of muscle strength, usually caused by an extreme emotional stimulus.

Basics of Epilepsy

Narcolepsy, obstructive sleep apnea, restless leg syndrome, periodic leg movements in sleep are disorders that are more common in patients with epilepsy.

Other movement disorders such as dystonia (abnormal tone) and **paroxysmal kinesigenic choreoathetosis (PKC)** can raise doubt of epilepsy. Dystonia can be intermittent. Seizures can present with stiffening and increased tone of the muscles. PKC is another disorder that presents in the first 2 decades of life and tends to remit with older age. It is much more common in boys than girls. It can be precipitated as the patient stands up from a sitting position. This disorder is characterized by abnormal dancelike, purposeless movements for few minutes. Several such episodes can be present in a day, at times more than one hundred a day. These episodes are easily treated with very low doses of antiepileptics.

paroxysmal kinesigenic choreoathetosis (PKC)

A rare and easily treatable movement disorder. It is characterized by recurrent, brief involuntary "distorted" movements of the body that are provoked by sudden movements.

4. What do you mean by breath-holding spasms?

Breath-holding spasms are common in children less than 2 years of age. These are very frequently confused with seizures. These are provoked by some emotional stimuli such as pain, emotional stress, temper tantrum, excessive crying, or fear. These generally subside within a minute. The duration of the events is almost the same as tonic and atonic seizures. Usually a good history and known triggers help differentiate the nature of these events. Provocation by pain, crying, anger, or other emotional stimuli provides clues to the diagnosis. Breath-holding spasms are classified into two types—pallid and cyanotic.

Cyanotic spells are characterized by cyanosis—the skin turns blue. The child holds his or her breath in expiration. The child's lips turn blue; the whole body can go stiff or become limp. Because of a lack of oxygen to the blood, the child's skin turns blue as well. Parents may notice a few jerking movements of the body if their child holds his breath for a long time. The child quickly returns to normal state after a brief gasp of air and may go to sleep after the episode. A careful history can tease out the difference between cyanotic spells and seizures.

Pallid syncope is also characterized by stiffening and a few jerks of the extremities. The eyes roll up, and the child becomes limp. The child does not turn blue, unlike with cyanotic spells. The child looks completely pale and becomes briefly unresponsive. Pallid syncope is the result of the heart coming to a standstill. This is called **asystole**. Pallid syncope is particularly common after falls or head injuries. **Table 3** depicts some common causes of loss of consciousness not related to seizures. An EEG in children with pallid syncope is normal. These episodes tend to resolve spontaneously by 4 years of age.

5. Can my child outgrow epilepsy?

Your child might outgrow epilepsy; there is always a possibility especially under certain circumstances. Various benign epilepsies of infancy and childhood are listed

cyanotic spells
Spells associated with fear, trauma, and emotional stress. A child stops breathing, turns blue, and may have a brief loss of consciousness.

pallid syncope
Often precipitated by trauma, a condition in which the child becomes limp and extremely pale with very brief loss of consciousness.

asystole
No electrical activity of the heart; the heart stops pumping.

Table 3 Common Causes of Syncope
• Vasovagal syncope: fear, pain, situational
• Syncopal episodes after meals, cough, urination, defecation (passing stools)
• Positional/orthostatic hypotension
• Heart-related or cardiac causes
• No discernible cause

in **Table 4**. Neonates and infants may have a seizure disorder that has a benign course. The chances of outgrowing epilepsy vary with different childhood epilepsy syndromes.

Healthy neonates (less than 28 days old) can have seizures in the first week of life, with peak onset on the second or third day of life. These can last up to 3 months of life. The child can turn blue. These seizures can last from a few seconds to 2 minutes. It is uncommon to see **generalized seizures** in neonates because the brain is still immature. Benign neonatal convulsions and benign neonatal sleep myoclonus epilepsies are seen in normal full-term infants with good apgar scores. These patients develop normally, have normal MRIs of the brain, but have only myoclonic seizures. One atypical feature is that myoclonic seizures tend to occur during drowsiness.

Other benign epilepsy **syndromes** such as **childhood absence** and juvenile absence epilepsies have very good prognosis, and those who have these conditions typically outgrow them.

Benign occipital epilepsy is another benign syndrome, which was first described by Henri Gastaut. The seizures are characterized by visual symptoms. An EEG

generalized seizure

Abnormal electrical activity occurring simultaneously from both sides of the brain.

syndrome

A combination of signs and/or symptoms occurring together indicating a particular disorder.

childhood absence epilepsy

Age-related benign generalized epilepsy with very brief clusters of absence seizures; these seizures are also referred to as petit mal seizures.

benign occipital epilepsy

One of the benign forms of epilepsy of childhood with partial seizures associated with visual auras.

Table 4   Benign Epilepsy Syndromes
• Benign familial neonatal convulsions
• Benign neonatal convulsions
• Benign infantile epilepsy
• Benign myoclonic epilepsy in infancy
• Benign rolandic epilepsy
• Childhood absence epilepsy (petit mal)
• Juvenile absence epilepsy (impulsive petit mal)
• Juvenile myoclonic epilepsy
• Benign occipital epilepsy
• Panayiotopoulos syndrome

shows spikes in the occipital areas when the child closes his or her eyes (**Figure 2**). This is called late-onset childhood epilepsy with occipital epilepsy. Remission occurs in about half of the patients within a couple of years after the onset. This syndrome could be confused with migraines as the two conditions may coexist. A child suffering from common migraine with visual auras can have the same presentation and EEG can show epilepsy brain waves. But the visual auras of migraines are followed by a bad headache, nausea, and/or vomiting and other family members with history of migraines.

Panayiotopoulos describes a syndrome characterized by vomiting during seizures, as well as periods of confusion, disorientation, and head and eye deviation. Seizures are prolonged and may meet the criteria of status epilepticus. However, this is classified under benign disorders.

Panayiotopoulos

A recently described benign form of epilepsy where seizures are characterized by nausea, retching, and vomiting. EEG shows abnormal epilepsy brain waves in the back of the head.

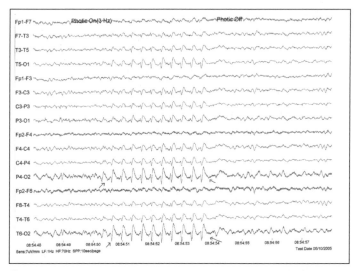

Figure 2
EEG showing occipital spikes (indicated by arrows) with maximal electrical field in O_2, O_1 ($O_2 > O_1$). *Source:* Reproduced from Singh A. 2006. *100 Questions and Answers About Epilepsy.* Sudbury, Massachusetts: Jones and Bartlett Publishers, LLC.

Benign psychomotor epilepsy starts typically between 2 and 9 years of age. Children can have chewing problems, swallowing movements, sweating, drooling, moaning, trouble speaking, abdominal pain, and loss of awareness in the level of consciousness during a typical seizure. These tend to last 1–2 minutes.

6. I have never seen anyone having a seizure. Can you explain to me what I should look for in my son?

The questions that follow should give you an idea of what to look for when you suspect your son is having a seizure:

- What time of the day do the events tend to occur?
- Does he have any warning signs? Does he give you a clue that a seizure is about to happen, or try to reach for help?
- Does he stare or freeze, stop doing an activity or stop interacting with the environment? Is there subtle or complete loss of consciousness? How long does he remain unresponsive?
- Does he stiffen his body?
- What do his arms or legs do? Do they stiffen or jerk, or first stiffen and then jerk? Or do they just start jerking without stiffening first? Does stiffness or jerking begin with the right or left side of the body and then spread to the other side?
- Does he lose his balance or fall?
- What do you see on your son's face? Do his eyes roll up?
- Do you see any facial or eye twitching?

Basics of Epilepsy

- Does he blink his eyes rapidly? Are there any abnormal mouth movements, such as chewing or lip-smacking movements?
- Does his face sweat? Are there changes in skin color—paleness, redness/flushed, or blueness?
- Is there any tongue biting or urinary **incontinence**? Does he have an urge to vomit or pass urine or stools during or after the seizure?
- Does he start breathing heavily?
- Does his head go to one side? Do his eyes or head go to one side in a jerky fashion?
- Has he suffered from any physical injury during apparent seizures?
- Have his teacher or friends at school reported any seizures since the last visit?
- What happens after the seizure or event? How long does he take to recuperate? Does he develop any weakness after the seizures? Is it generalized fatigue? Is there any loss of strength or sensations on one side or the other, or are there visual or hearing deficits?

It is important to keep a log for any typical or atypical episodes. These should be recorded in a **seizure diary** or **seizure calendar**. You should bring this diary when you see your son's **neurologist** or **epileptologist**. This tells your doctor how many events or seizures occurred since the last visit. Your physician can compare the frequency of events since the last follow-up. Sometimes, there may be changes in the severity (less or more intense) of the seizures even if there is no significant change in the frequency. The duration of the seizures helps the physician decide if you need to give your son emergency medicine. Let your son's physician know if you think there are any

incontinence
Involuntary urination.

seizure diary
A diary maintained by the patient, parent, or a caregiver where the frequency of seizures, duration, and patient behavior during the seizures are recorded.

seizure calendar
A calendar maintained by the patient, parent, or a caregiver where patient marks the number of different seizure type(s). A physician can judge the frequency of the seizure.

neurologist
A physician who specializes in conditions of the nervous system.

epileptologist
A neurologist who specializes in epilepsy.

provoking factors for seizures. Some seizures are provoked by obvious external stimuli. You can write some footnotes if you think the seizure was provoked. These help your son's physician to make a decision whether the medication dosages need to be increased or not. Common causes of seizure provocation are as follows:

- Missed medications
- Sleep deprivation
- Alcohol provocation
- Viral or other physical illness/physical stress
- Vomiting/diarrhea (probably did not absorb medications)
- Emotional stress (positive or negative)

Seizures are broadly classified into two categories—partial or generalized. Features described by the families or the patient help physicians to correctly classify the seizure type. **Table 5** lists the common seizure types in two broad categories of epilepsy.

7. Are seizures harmful to my child's developing brain?

Experimental studies on animals have tried to answer this question for many decades. An immature brain is more susceptible to seizures. The majority of seizures do not cause any long-term sequelae. That being said, brain development is affected by the frequency and severity of seizures. A child's brain is immature at the time of birth and continues to lay down important neuronal networks and thereby continues to mature. The brain of a fetus grows at an astonishing rate and can add up to 250,000

Basics of Epilepsy

Table 5 Classification of Seizures

Generalized seizures
- Absence (petit mal)
- Myoclonic (sudden jerks)
- Tonic-clonic
- Tonic
- Clonic

Partial seizures
- Simple partial seizures
- Complex partial seizures
- Complex partial with secondary generalization

Unclassified

---

neurons every minute; this phenomenon is called **proliferation**. Insignificant or unused brain connections get pruned by a process called programmed cell death or **apoptosis**. Maturation of neurons and development of synapses among neurons continues after birth. The neuron cells migrate from one part to the other parts of the brain. The brain differentiates into gray and white matter. Gray looks gray to the naked eye and is the main processing center. The communication networks or synapses (means by which cells communicate with each other) are formed in the adjacent areas as well as between the two hemispheres. Poorly controlled seizures can have deleterious effects on the proper migration or synaptogenesis of neurons. Myelin formation is an important part of brain development. Myelin is a white fatty substance that envelops the axons and provides insulation to brain pathways. Myelin also helps faster transmission of impulses from one neuron to another. This process is called **myelination** and is very important for laying down of subcortical networks in the brain. This forms the white matter in the brain,

proliferation

A rapid increase or growth.

apoptosis

Programmed cell death.

myelination

Process of formation of myelin around the nerve fibers.

17

which looks white to the naked eye. By age 2, 80% of the adult brain is formed; and by age 6, 95% of the adult brain is formed. Girls' brains reach their maximum size earlier than boys, maturing at 11.5 years and 14.5 years, respectively. Certain parts of the brain, such as prefrontal lobes, centers that are important for planning, reasoning, impulse control, judgment, problem solving, social interactions, and so forth, may not mature until late in the teenage years or in the twenties.

There is an old aphorism by William Gowers that says, "Seizures beget seizures." Scientists have been trying to determine whether seizures are harmful to developing brains in experimental animal models and in humans as physicians strive hard to achieve seizure freedom in their clinical practices. Scientists question whether the brain's electrical networks get strengthened as seizures continue to occur. Whether ongoing seizures lower the threshold of recurrence in a child or increase the risk of recurrence is an area of ongoing research. Cognitive problems, behavioral problems, and learning difficulties have been well recognized in children with epilepsy. Possible reasons for learning disabilities include:

- Difficulty with working memory or transferring information from short-term to long-term memory.
- Left brain dysfunction, which affects language and verbal memory.
- Right brain dysfunction, which results in decreased visuospatial memory (patients might get lost or face difficulty following directions).
- Medications can affect cognition.
- Abnormalities on the EEG.

- Subclinical seizures (EEG showing seizures without any obvious change in the behavior).

Medically refractory seizures can lead to cognitive decline and behavioral and psychiatric problems. This argument makes a case for early surgical intervention in children who do not respond to medical intervention.

Basics of Epilepsy

PART TWO

Classification of Seizures

What are febrile seizures?

My son has jaw jerks when he reads.
When he stops reading, he feels better.
Can reading or other stimuli trigger seizures?

What are infantile spasms?

More ...

8. What are febrile seizures?

Febrile seizure occurs in relation to high fever in infants from 6 months to children 4 years of age. On average, 33% of children who have had a single febrile seizure have at least one recurrence. Sometimes, febrile seizures run in families. The parents, siblings, or first cousins in the family might be affected. Febrile seizures can be of two kinds—simple and complex. A **simple febrile seizure** lasts for 1–2 minutes. The seizure type usually has generalized tonic-clonic features without any focal features such as head or eyes turning to one side or involvement of one side of the body more than the other.

On the contrary, a **complex febrile seizure** may show focal or partial features such as head or eyes deviation to one side. It may last for longer than 1–2 minutes. There could be asymmetric involvement of the body. Complex febrile seizures tend to recur within 24 hours.

Most of the febrile seizures are self-limited and are genetically predetermined. Less than 10% of all febrile seizures recur or are severe. Less than 5% of those with febrile seizures develop epilepsy. Febrile seizures are associated with a higher risk of developing medically refractory seizures later in life, though the risk is small. The risk of developing chronic epilepsy is higher if seizures are prolonged, if they include focal features, or if they recur within 24 hours. There is a delay before residual epilepsy is recognized. Children may remain seizure free for many years before the recurrence. They commonly develop complex partial seizures. The **temporal lobe** in the brain gets involved. An MRI done on the brain of one of these patients shows abnormality called **mesial temporal sclerosis**. Sclerosis means scar;

simple febrile seizure

Seizure occurring in relation to a high fever; usually a brief, grand mal seizure without any focal features.

complex febrile seizure

Seizure occurring in relation to high fever, usually prolonged, and may show asymmetric involvement of the body or focal features clinically.

temporal lobe

The part of the brain that is involved in speech, language, memory, and the perception of smell and taste.

mesial temporal sclerosis

Subtle scar seen in the temporal lobes in patients with temporal lobe epilepsy due to neuronal loss.

this is projected as a linear abnormal signal (example seen in **Figure 3**) involving the most medial structures of the temporal lobe, namely the **hippocampus** and **amygdala**. The finding of mesial temporal sclerosis is not confined to patients with febrile seizures. Other risk factors such as head trauma, brain infections, or prolonged seizures (status epilepticus) can cause similar findings on the MRI. If seizures are refractory to more than two or three antiepileptics, then presurgical evaluation should be done to see if the patient is a good surgical candidate for one of the epilepsy surgeries (see Part Seven).

hippocampus

Part of the temporal lobe of the brain that is involved in memory consolidation.

amygdala

Part of the temporal lobe involved in human emotions.

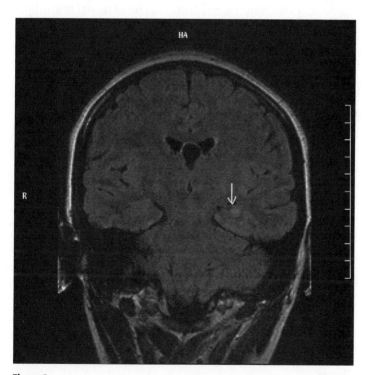

Figure 3
Left mesial hippocampal sclerosis. *Source:* Reproduced from Singh A. 2006. *100 Questions and Answers About Epilepsy.* Sudbury, Massachusetts: Jones and Bartlett Publishers, LLC.

9. My son has jaw jerks when he reads. When he stops reading, he feels better. Can reading or other stimuli trigger seizures?

Various external stimuli can trigger seizures. This is called **reflex epilepsy**. Symptoms that you just described are typical of one of the types of reflex epilepsy called **primary reading epilepsy**. It is a rare disorder. In patients with reading epilepsy, reading can cause seizures. It starts initially with jaw jerks and jaw discomfort. If the patient continues to read, the jaw jerks may evolve into a tonic-clonic seizure. These seizures can be averted by stopping reading. The frequency of the seizures depends on the duration and complexity of reading. The triggering factors can be external stimuli or rarely even internal mental processes (**Figure 4**).

Most reflex epilepsies are really rare syndromes. Most of these are named after the trigger factors causing seizures. These disorders may have onset during childhood or adolescence. Flashes of light at particular fre-

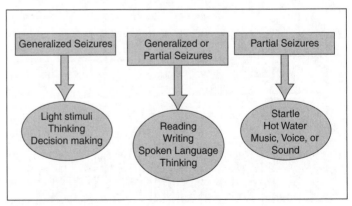

Figure 4

Reflex epilepsy syndromes related to various extraneous stimuli. *Source:* Reproduced from Singh A. 2006. *100 Questions and Answers About Epilepsy.* Sudbury, Massachusetts: Jones and Bartlett Publishers, LLC.

quencies can trigger epilepsy. This is called **photosensitive epilepsy**. About 30% of generalized epilepsies exhibit this phenomenon of **photosensitivity**. Patients are found to be sensitive to certain frequencies or wave patterns of light. Patients may find flickering sun glare along a tree-lined road as one of the triggers. Prolonged exposure to computers, animated cartoon programs, television, or video or electronic screen games can trigger seizures. Particular visual patterns such as alternating or oscillating black and white patterns could provoke seizures as well.

Certain tones of music notes can trigger seizures. This is called **musicogenic epilepsy**. Patients with this condition tend to avoid certain notes of music to avoid seizures. Language, speech, and auditory stimuli can trigger seizures. There are reported cases of seizures triggered by listening to someone's voice or a particular song. Complex decision making such as tough political decisions, deep thinking, mental processes, and arithmetic exercises could provoke seizures.

Tooth brushing, walking, and answering the telephone have been identified as other rare reflex epilepsies. **Eating epilepsy** is triggered by sight or smell of food. The seizures may occur at the beginning of eating a meal or after eating meals. Hot water has been a trigger for reflex seizures in some patients. **Hot water epilepsy** is more common in Southern India. Other stimuli like light touch or tapping may be associated with reflex seizures.

Most of the reflex epilepsies are easy to control, and seizures are rare. Patients learn how to work around trigger factors and by doing so avoid seizures.

photosensitive epilepsy
A form of epilepsy in which seizures are triggered by flickering or flashing light at particular frequencies.

photosensitivity
Situation in which seizures are triggered by lights flashing or flickering at particular frequencies and, sometimes, by certain geometric shapes or patterns.

musicogenic epilepsy
A kind of reflex epilepsy where seizures are precipitated by listening to music.

eating epilepsy
A rare form of reflex epilepsy that is precipitated by eating.

hot water epilepsy
One of the rare forms of reflex epilepsy caused by bathing with hot water. This is more common in southern parts of India.

Classification of Seizures

10. What are infantile spasms?

infantile spasms (IS)

Clusters of rapid jerks followed by stiffening or jackknife movements.

Infantile spasms (IS) are very brief, rapid, tonic contractions of the trunk and limbs; these can last 5–10 seconds, constituting about 2% of childhood epilepsies. William West described these in 1841. Males are slightly more affected than the females. Peak age of onset is 4–6 months. These tend to occur in clusters and are very common before sleep or upon awakening. These may be provoked by touch. Each cluster can have dozens or up to hundreds of infantile spasms per day and can last 10–15 minutes. Spasms can resemble a startle response in an infant. Spasms can be flexors, extensors, or mixed. During flexor spasms, the hands acquire a self-hugging position. The neck or body can bend forward, or the arms may bend at the elbow. The neck may suddenly move backward and the arms or legs may straighten. Extensor spasms are characterized by arms that thrash backwards. Mixed spasms are the most common. In other kinds, the head may just suddenly thrust forward, or it could be more subtle head nods.

Patients with infantile spasms show a very unique pattern during seizures and in between seizures.

Patients with infantile spasms show a very unique pattern during seizures and in between seizures. In between the spasms, these patients may have a very high voltage, chaotic EEG background lacking any organization, with multiple spikes, sharps, and slow waves (see Question 21 for a discussion of EEGs). This pattern is called **hypsarrhythmia**. During the spasms, the EEG shows flattening of the very abnormal background for few seconds. This is called **electrodecremental response**.

hypsarrhythmia

A distinctive EEG pattern associated with infantile spasms.

electrodecremental response

Change in the EEG background during an intantile spasm.

West syndrome

A syndrome characterized by infantile spasms, mental retardation, and a specific EEG pattern (hypsarrhthymia).

The infantile spasms may be associated with mental retardation or developmental delay. This triad of infantile spasms, hypsarrythmia, and developmental delay is clinically recognized as **West syndrome**.

Some patients with infantile spasms have a positive family history. An MRI of the brain may not show any structural abnormality. Patients may have a cryptogenic cause, where the cause is suspected but is hidden (cryptic). Cryptogenic causes account for about 40% of the cases of infantile spasms. Other children may have more obvious causes, such as birth trauma, brain hypoxia/**anoxia,** or brain hemorrhages; these are called symptomatic cases. Symptomatic cases account for about 60% of the cases. **Table 6** classifies different causes of infantile spasms.

There could be other more obvious cases where the physician suspects these syndromes by abnormal skin manifestations noted on exam. These are called **neurocutaneous syndromes** (neuro = neurological; cutaneous = skin). There are three common neurocutaneous syndromes, which are:

1. **Tuberous sclerosis** (80–90% have seizures)
2. **Neurofibromatosis** (3–5%)
3. **Sturge-Weber syndrome** (90%)

Infantile spasms may be associated with other seizure types such as complex partial, tonic, or clonic seizures.

anoxia
A lack of oxygen.

neurocutaneous syndromes
Genetic disorders where there is involvement of the skin along with abnormal growth of tumors in various parts of the body and central nervous system.

tuberous sclerosis
A neurological condition associated with seizures, mental retardation, and skin lesions.

neurofibromatosis
One of the most common neurocutaenous syndromes.

Sturge-Weber syndrome
A congenital disease present at birth and characterized by a facial birthmark or port-wine stain (reddish brown or pink discoloration of the face).

Table 6 Causes of Infantile Spasms

Symptomatic
Before birth: Tuberous sclerosis, Down syndrome, trauma, Sturge-Weber syndrome
Around birth: Lack of oxygen or blood flow to the brain, brain infections, trauma, brain hemorrhages
After birth: Metabolic and genetic disorders, pyridoxine dependency, biotinidase deficiency, mitochondrial disorders, degenerative diseases, trauma

Cryptogenic: No discernible cause but underlying brain insult is suspected

Idiopathic: No underlying disorder is suspected, MRI of the brain and neurological examination normal

11. My daughter has been inattentive at school; her teachers have been complaining that she has been daydreaming a lot. I noticed her staring at the dinner table, and she did not respond to me when I called her name. Can she be having seizures?

absence seizure

Brief episode of staring lasting a few seconds.

Your daughter may have what we call **absence seizures**. This seizure disorder may go undiagnosed for a long time. Children have brief staring spells that could be extremely subtle. Typical absence seizures tend to last 5–10 seconds. Kids can have 10–100 absence seizures a day. Children have frequent staring spells and are often misdiagnosed as being less attentive. Parents may hear from a child's teacher that the child is always in a dreamy state. Children usually do not have a clue that their seizures are occurring. These children do not get any preceding aura or any symptoms afterwards. Your daughter may notice that she missed part of a conversation. Staring spells are easily precipitated by deep breathing exercises. A pediatrician can confirm the diagnosis of absence epilepsy in his or her office by asking your daughter to breathe into a paper bag, thus capturing the typical staring spells. The EEG can confirm the diagnosis. Hyperventilation (deep breathing exercises) during the EEG test should be included if absence seizures are suspected.

The peak age of onset is 6–7 years of age. Girls are affected more than boys. Children with absence seizures are developmentally normal. The abnormality on the EEG may be more obvious when the child is asked to start deep breathing. Absence status (prolonged, continuous absence seizures lasting more than 30 minutes) is seen in 10% of children who have absence seizures.

It is believed that the thalamus is the generator of generalized epilepsy. Absence seizures can be confused with partial seizures. Absences, unlike partial seizures, start from both parts of the brain and are classified under generalized epilepsies. It is important to make a correct diagnosis, as wrong selection of medications can worsen absence seizures. Certain drugs such as carbamazepine, sabril, gabitril, and phenytoin may worsen absences.

Absence seizures can be very subtle. Since these seizures start diffusely from both sides of the brain, the patient has no clue he or she had a seizure. Patient resumes ongoing activity after a very brief pause as if nothing happened and does not go into a postictal state of sleepiness, confusion, or disorientation. Patients usually cannot tell they had a seizure and are unable to keep a count of their own seizures. Families and teachers miss it as well. Teachers misdiagnose the problem, saying that the student is less attentive in the classroom. Parents may name the problem *daydreaming*.

Absence seizures are characterized by a very specific EEG pattern called 3-Hertz (Hz) spike and wave activity. Hertz is a unit of frequency and is measured per second. So in a 3-Hz spike and wave, in one second, the epilepsy brain waves occur three times. This pattern is very regular and may occur in bursts. The burst can last for a variable length of time. It is understandable that frequent or longer bursts can be associated with learning problems. Patients with longer bursts are able to recognize that they probably had a seizure as they miss a segment of conversation or notice they have brief lapses of time loss. If parents notice these events, the child should have the EEG done. Hyperventilation can induce one of the typical events. If absence seizures are suspected, a seizure can be induced by telling the patient to do deep breathing in a paper bag. The diagnosis can be made if a typical staring spell is witnessed during hyperventilation and confirmed by a typical 3-Hz spike and wave pattern on the EEG. A prolonged absence seizure is classified as absence status epilepticus, which is a seizure lasting for more than 30 minutes; however, such a sesizure can last for several hours or even days. The absence status can terminate as a grand mal seizure. Prolonged absence status indicates failure of seizure-terminating mechanisms of the brain.

There are two kinds of absence seizures—**typical** and **atypical**. Typical absences are characterized by abrupt, brief staring, behavioral arrest, and impaired consciousness. Patients might have few eye blinks. Sometimes the eye blinks are more repetitive.

Atypical absences are characterized by staring, eye blinking, slight jerking of the arms, and some lip smacking. There could be changes in the postural tone. There could be nodding of the head. These last longer than the typical absences, commonly lasting longer than 10 seconds (mean 5–30 seconds). These have some overlapping features of complex partial seizures. Atypical absences occur in children with developmental and cognitive delays. At times, it is hard to distinguish these from their usual behavior. Other seizure types associated with atypical absences are atonic seizures, **astatic seizures** or tonic seizures described in other sections of the book. The EEG in atypical absences is characterized by **slow spike and slow waves** (frequency less than 2.5 Hz). The typical absence has a higher frequency spike and slow wave more than 2.5 Hz. Motor and behavioral phenomena are more common with atypical absences.

typical absence

Brief staring and behavioral arrest for 5–10 seconds with 3 Hz spike and wave pattern on the EEG.

atypical absence

A seizure type characterized by staring spells which may be associated with eye blinking, strange hand movements, or lip smacking, and can be confused with complex partial seizures.

astatic seizures

Partial or complete loss of muscle tone causing inability to stand, usually with clear consciousness.

slow spike and slow waves

In generalized epilepsies, some waves are recognized by their shape and form, and by the frequency. Slow spike and wave is the irregular burst of spike and slow wave of frequency less than 2.5 hertz. This pattern is seen in Lennox-Gastaut syndrome.

Spasm-like frequent movements of the eyes can be seen initially followed by absences. This is called eyelid myoclonia. The eyeballs can roll up. Eyelid myoclonia can be induced by intermittent photic stimulation and eye closure. The combination of eyelid myoclonia and absences is referred to as **Jeavons syndrome**. Absence seizures can be seen with myoclonic and tonic-clonic seizures. Absence seizures are seen in several age-related epilepsy syndromes such as childhood absence epilepsy, juvenile absence epilepsy, and juvenile myoclonic epilepsy. Juvenile myoclonic epilepsy has two other seizure types in addition to absence seizures— myoclonic and tonic-clonic. Absences alone can respond well to ethosuximide (Zarontin). When there are other seizure types in addition to absences, then other broad-spectrum antiepileptics such as divalproex sodium (Depakote), lamotrigine (Lamictal) and topiramate (Topamax), or zonisamide (Zonegran) should be tried.

Juvenile absence epilepsy is also characterized by staring spells. The peak age of onset is around 10–12 years. The staring spells are not as frequent as in childhood absence, but they tend to last longer. There is more subtle change in the level of consciousness. Children can have other seizure types such as tonic-clonic seizures and myoclonic.

Benign focal epilepsy of childhood is also called **benign rolandic epilepsy**. This is the most common kind of benign focal epilepsy. Children with this type of epilepsy have normal intelligence. They attend regular schools and have normal neurologic examinations. This is one of the epilepsy syndromes in which the child looks healthy, but the EEG looks sick. An EEG shows very frequent

Classification of Seizures

Jeavons syndrome
Absence seizures and myoclonic movements of the eyelids.

juvenile absence epilepsy
Primarily absence seizures with onset near puberty; myoclonic and grand mal seizures are also seen.

benign rolandic epilepsy
A benign epilepsy syndrome, categorized as partial epilepsy; patients have nocturnal focal seizures with very abnormal EEG, normal MRI of the brain, and normal neurological exam.

abnormal epileptiform waves, especially when the child goes to sleep. Parents notice rare seizures in the night-time; they report their children look scared, have facial twitching, and drool. Rarely do they have tonic-clonic seizures. This syndrome usually presents at 8–9 years of age. Children do not have any long-term sequelae. The seizures are easily controlled by low doses of antiepileptic medications. Children have remissions in the second decade of life. Rarely, all three seizure types (absence, myoclonic, and tonic-clonic) may persist and represent the other spectrum, called **juvenile myoclonic epilepsy**. **Figure 5** depicts a typical burst of spikes, polyspikes, and slow waves on light stimulation.

juvenile myoclonic epilepsy

A syndrome with onset during teenage years, characterized by absence, tonic-clonic, and myoclonic seizures.

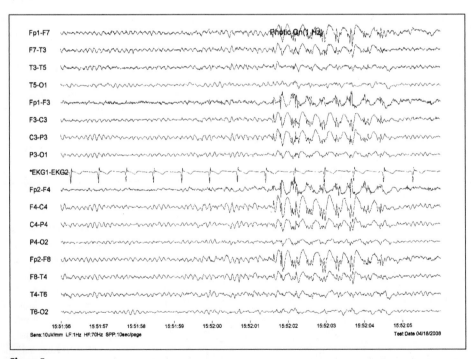

Figure 5
EEG in juvenile myoclonic epilepsy, activated by photic stimulation, shows abnormal discharges called spike and slow wave.

Atypical absences can have other associated features such as eye blinking, mouth movements, upward eye rotation, and hand movements. These can be confused with complex partial seizures. Atypical absences are seen in patients with developmental delays and complex neurological syndromes.

12. My child has brief jerking movements during sleep and when he wakes up. These movements are very brief, and he does not lose consciousness. What are these?

These sound like and could be **myoclonic seizures**. Myoclonus is brief, sudden contraction of the large group of muscles, just for a split second. These need to be differentiated from a very common phenomenon experienced by most of us as we fall asleep. This is called physiologic myoclonus of sleep. Another common example of myoclonus, in normal individuals, is hiccups due to irritation of one of the muscles of respiration. In myoclonus, the arms are more commonly involved than the legs. Both sides of the body get involved. Myoclonus can occur at any age starting from infancy to old age. Myoclonus is also seen in advanced kidney and liver diseases or can be the result of lack of oxygen to the brain. Insults around the time of birth such as brain anoxia, brain maldevelopment, or inborn errors of metabolism could be the cause of myoclonus. Myoclonus has been associated with various benign and catastrophic and progressive epilepsy syndromes and other neurodegenerative diseases of the brain, as listed in **Table 7**.

Juvenile myoclonic epilepsy is one of the genetically inherited epilepsies associated with myoclonic seizures, absence seizures, and tonic-clonic seizures. Myoclonus

myoclonic seizures
Generalized seizures with brief jerks of the whole body or a part of the body.

Classification of Seizures

Table 7 Epilepsy Syndromes Associated with Myoclonic Seizures
Benign myoclonic epilepsy of infancy
GEFS+*
Eyelid myoclonia with absences
Ohtahara syndrome
Lennox-Gastaut syndrome
Lafora disease
Neuronal ceroid lipofuschinosis
Juvenile myoclonic epilepsy

*GEFS+: Generalized epilepsy with febrile seizures plus

occurs during morning hours and can precede a grand mal seizure. This syndrome typically sets in during teenage years; children may drop objects from their hands or lose balance if myoclonic seizures involve arms or legs respectively. Jerks or twitches might not be so obvious, but the patient would complain of leg or arm jumps. Myoclonic seizures can be associated with other seizure types such as atonic, atypical absence, tonic, and partial seizures. **Progressive myoclonic epilepsy (PME)** may be associated with myoclonic and generalized tonic-clonic seizures. Other symptoms such as loss of memory, blindness, trouble walking, and strokes can be seen in patients with PME. PMEs are suspected based on the clinical features. Diagnostic testing such as brain MRI, EEG, thorough eye examination, ultrasound of the heart, skin biopsy, or muscle biopsy may be necessary to reach a conclusive diagnosis. Patients with PME may present with prolonged myoclonic seizures lasting more than 30 minutes, which is called **myoclonic status**.

progressive myoclonic epilepsy (PME)

A neurological condition characterized by myoclonic and grand mal seizures, as well as developmental delays. It may have visual, memory, or balance problems.

myoclonic status

Continuous myoclonic jerks lasting more than 30 minutes.

drop attack

A sudden loss of muscle tone resulting in falls and physical injuries.

akinetic seizure

Seizure characterized by brief limping of body and loss of consciousness.

13. My child suddenly drops his head or becomes limp and falls on the ground, resulting in head traumas. What can be done?

Your description of events raises concerns about what we call **drop attacks**, **akinetic seizures**, or **atonic**

seizures, which occur when a child suddenly loses body tone. In the past, these were also referred to as astatic or static seizures. Neuroscientists believe that there are specific negative motor areas in our brains that may be involved in atonic seizures. Atonic seizures can be generalized or focal. The patient has no premonitory symptoms if these are generalized in onset. The loss in body tone can be complete or partial. It may be limited to extremities, jaw, or head muscles. If limited to the head, children would suddenly drop their head—usually forward. When the loss of body tone is complete, the child is prone to sudden falls. I advise my patients with drop attacks to wear a helmet for their safety.

Atonic seizures need to be differentiated from **tonic seizures**, in which a sudden muscle contraction can result in a fall. Myoclonic seizures and myoclonic astatic seizures can cause falls as well. Focal atonic seizures commonly originate from the **frontal lobe**. The **motor cortex** (cortex involved in the movements of our different body parts) is located in the frontal lobes. Focal atonic seizures may be associated with temporary weakness or paralysis of the limbs.

Negative myoclonus is another abrupt event responsible for falling seizures. Nonneurological causes such as changes in the blood pressure or heart rhythm resulting in falls should be excluded as well. **Video EEG** can be particularly helpful in understanding the nature of these attacks.

Atonic seizures start during childhood and are extremely brief, lasting up to 15 seconds. Prolonged atonic seizures last up to 1 minute. Loss of consciousness is frequently seen with prolonged atonic seizures.

atonic seizure
Generalized seizure causing sudden loss of muscle tone resulting in falls to the ground.

tonic seizures
Generalized seizures, in which a person's body becomes stiff, and he or she may fall backward.

frontal lobe
The part of the brain that is involved in movement and some aspects of thought, judgment initiation, and abstract thinking.

motor cortex
Part of the brain that controls voluntary movements.

negative myoclonus
Sudden involuntary relaxation of a muscle, rather than a contraction.

video EEG
A test involving simultaneous EEG and video recording.

Lennox-Gastaut syndrome

A severe form of epilepsy that usually begins in early childhood and is characterized by frequent seizures of multiple types causing falls and injuries, mental impairment, and a particular brain wave pattern (a slow spike-and-wave pattern).

Doose syndrome

A rare disorder with frequent and sudden drop attacks, violent myoclonic jerks, or abrupt loss of muscular tone (e.g., astatic seizures).

ketogenic diet

A high-fat diet that is sometimes used to treat severe epilepsy in children.

corpus callosotomy

Disconnection of corpus callosum (*see* corpus callosum).

partial epilepsy

Epilepsy originating from a part of the cortex.

generalized epilepsy

Epilepsy characterized by different seizure types, such as tonic-clonic, clonic, tonic, absence, or myoclonic seizures.

reticular activating system

The part of the brain that plays an important role in arousal and alertness.

Children may have brain damage, developmental delays, or mental retardation. Atonic seizures are seen with specific epileptic syndromes such as **Lennox-Gastaut syndrome** and **Doose syndrome**. Seizures may be hard to control with AEDs. Divalproex sodium, lamotrigine, topiramate, zonisamide, levetiracetam (Keppra), and felbamate (Felbatol) could be useful to treat atonic seizures. A **ketogenic diet** is another alternative. Children who fail medical therapy and continue to have frequent falls should be referred for brain surgery called **corpus callosotomy**.

14. What is generalized epilepsy?

There are two broad classifications of epilepsy—**partial** and **generalized**. By generalized, we mean that seizures start from both hemispheres. Because of the diffuse onset of the seizure, consciousness is lost right from the beginning. Patients with generalized epilepsy do not get any warning and cannot tell if they had a seizure. They wake up from a generalized tonic-clonic seizure confused and disoriented, not knowing what happened to them. Some patients can tell they had a seizure based on their previous experiences or if they bruised or injured themselves or woke up with a pool of blood or bit their tongue.

On the contrary, partial epilepsy has a focal onset. A focal seizure in one part of the brain can spread to both hemispheres. The brain is important for consciousness. There are areas in the brain that make up the **reticular activating system**, which is important for consciousness. When both hemispheres get involved in a seizure, consciousness is lost. Patients with partial seizures can recall their aura or can discuss some of the symptoms they experience before they got confused or lost their consciousness. This aura could last a few seconds to a few minutes. It is very important to make a distinction between partial and generalized epilepsy. This distinction can usually be made on the basis of clinical history and EEG pattern. Generalized epilepsy seems to originate from **thalamus-cortical network**. The thalamus is an important part of the brain responsible for pain perception. Thalamocortical pathways are important for typical EEG patterns seen during sleep called **sleep spindles**.

Generalized epilepsies tend to begin at an earlier age and are believed to have a genetic basis. Generalized epilepsies have different seizure types. Absence, clonic, tonic, myoclonic, and tonic-clonic seizures are different subcategories of generalized seizures. However, the pattern of inheritance is complex. Generalized epilepsies can be divided into three types:

1. *Idiopathic* (no apparent cause)
2. *Cryptogenic* (there is a likely cause that could not be identified; **cryptic** = hidden)
3. *Symptomatic* (cause has been identified, such as remote insult during birth, inborn errors of metabolism, genetic or chromosomal abnormalities)

Patients with **idiopathic epilepsy** have normal development, normal neurological examination, and normal MRI. However, their EEGs show a signature suggestive of generalized epilepsy. This EEG pattern is called **spikes** and slow wave. A spike signifies excitation. This is followed by a slow wave, which signifies inhibition. This pattern is easy to identify and can come in **bursts** lasting a few milliseconds or seconds. A burst of more than 3 seconds can produce a clinical symptom.

thalamus-cortical network

Important network system in the brain that plays a major role in the spread of seizures and connects the thalamus to the cortex or vice versa.

sleep spindles

A brain activity that happens during sleep. Sleep is divided into 4 stages, 1–4. Sleep spindles are seen during stage 1 and stage 2 sleep.

cryptic

Hidden.

idiopathic epilepsy

Epilepsy in which the cause of the condition is not known but genetic factors are believed to be involved.

spike

Narrow-based waves that have high amplitude. These are recorded from close to the seizure focus and are narrower shaped, lasting 20–70 milliseconds.

bursts

A sudden appearance of abnormal electrical discharges in the brain lasting milliseconds, seconds, or minutes.

Classification of Seizures

Examples of idiopathic generalized epilepsy include childhood absence, juvenile absence, juvenile myoclonic epilepsy, and epilepsy with grand-mal seizures on awakening. Common examples of symptomatic or cryptogenic generalized epilepsies include West syndrome and Lennox-Gastaut syndrome. Generalized epilepsies have different seizure types. Absence, clonic, tonic, myoclonic, and tonic-clonic seizures are different subcategories of generalized seizures. EEG patterns are unique to various generalized seizure types and syndromes. **Table 8** shows the patterns of various types of epilepsy syndrome.

15. My child started having seizures right after birth. What could cause them?

These are called neonatal seizures. Neonate is the term used for the first 28 days of life. Sometimes, abnormal movements or seizures may be reported by the mother in utero, before the child is born. One such example is seizures related to **pyridoxine** (vitamin B_6) dependency. Neonatal seizures are commonly associated with the following conditions:

pyridoxine

Vitamin B_6.

Table 8 EEG Patterns in Generalized Epilepsies	
Type of epilepsy	EEG pattern
Childhood absence epilepsy	Regular 3–3.5 Hz* spike and slow wave with anterior predominance
Juvenile absence epilepsy	Same as above
Atypical absence	Slow (less than 2.5 Hz*) spike and slow wave
Juvenile myoclonic epilepsy	Irregular faster (4–6 Hz*) spikes and polyspikes and slow waves
Tonic	Low amplitude, fast activity

*Hz indicates hertz, which is a unit of frequency; one Hz is equal to one cycle per second

- Genetic or inborn disorders of metabolism
- Trauma sustained at birth (prolonged labor, difficult delivery, forceps delivery)
- Decreased blood (**ischemia**) or oxygen (**hypoxia**) supply to the brain
- Brain infection
- Brain hemorrhage, either spontaneous or induced by difficult birth
- Drug withdrawal
- Electrolyte abnormalities (low glucose, low calcium, acidosis, high ammonia)
- Strokes suffered in utero

There are both benign and catastrophic age-related epilepsy syndromes presenting in the neonatal life in which seizures can be reported as early as during the first few days of life. Metabolic disorders of fat, carbohydrates, and protein metabolism tend to present with seizures when the neonate is fed with milk. Neonates do not have generalized seizures, as their immature brains lack the synapses or "networking." Neonates manifest the following four types of seizures:

1. **Clonic seizures**: This type of seizure is a rhythmic contraction and relaxation of different muscle groups. This is the most common seizure type in neonates.
2. **Tonic seizures:** This type of seizure is characterized by stiffening of part of the lower or upper extremities or whole body without any jerking movements; it tends to last 20–30 seconds. Premature infants are more prone to exhibit this seizure type.
3. **Myoclonic seizures**: This type of seizure is characterized by rapid, brief jerking movements of a

ischemia

The prolonged lack of blood supply to the brain.

hypoxia

The prolonged lack of oxygen to the brain.

Neonates do not have generalized seizures, as their immature brains lack the synapses or "networking."

clonic seizure

Epileptic seizure characterized by jerking movements that involve muscles on both sides of the body.

subtle seizures

Seen in premature or mature neonates (less than 4 weeks old). Brief blinking, staring, tongue or mouth movements, pedaling, stiffening of the limbs, or just eye deviation can represent subtle seizures.

automatisms

Automatic or purposeless movements—typically occurring during a complex partial seizure—lip smacking, rearranging objects, chewing or swallowing movements, fumbling with clothing, and undressing.

autonomic neurons

Brain nerve cells that control those functions that are not controlled voluntarily, such as heart rate, contractions of the intestine, or sweat production.

fifth-day fits

These usually start on day 2 or 3 of life in otherwise healthy babies.

benign familial neonatal convulsions (BFNC)

Inherited form of epilepsy that manifests in the first week of life. Newborns suffer from tonic-clonic seizures.

mutation

Changes in the genetic material.

muscle group—usually large muscle groups such as shoulder or hip flexors.

4. **Subtle seizures**: As the name suggests, this seizure type can be more subtle. Parents may report chewing movements, eye deviation, or jerking movements. Other manifestations can be strange bicycling movements or other purposeless movements of the hands called **automatisms**. **Autonomic neurons** can get involved during seizures. Autonomic neurons are neurons that are not under conscious control. These neurons regulate heart activity, blood vessels, intestines, and various glands. Changes in the heart rate or blood pressure and sudden, brief changes in the breathing pattern (apnea) are some of the autonomic manifestations of subtle seizures.

There are few benign epilepsy syndromes seen in neonates. One such example is the benign neonatal myoclonus of sleep. Another benign syndrome is known as **fifth-day fits**, which manifest in the first week of life. They are characterized by brief clonic movements and apnea but carry an excellent prognosis. These seizures have no long-term sequelae, but about 0.5% of children go on to develop epilepsy at a later stage in life. At times, these children receive treatment, as these seizures tend to recur after 1–2 days. These children do not have a family history of seizures.

Benign familial neonatal convulsions is another benign epilepsy syndrome that is caused by a genetic defect or a change in a gene called a **mutation**. The gene defect is in the potassium channels. Potassium helps stabilize the cell membranes. There is usually a family history of seizures either in the neonatal period or a history of later epilepsy. The majority of neonates who develop seizures typically do so on the second or third day of life. This syndrome carries a benign prognosis. Association with febrile seizures and later epilepsy has been reported.

There is a mushrooming of literature on the effects of seizures on the developing brain and how a child's brain is different from an adult's. Researchers are trying to understand how neonatal seizures alter the neuronal synapses and have effects on cognition.

16. How is frontal lobe epilepsy different from temporal lobe epilepsy?

Frontal lobe epilepsy is the second most common epilepsy; temporal lobe epilepsy is the most common. The two frontal lobes, right and left, are connected to each other through a white compact structure called **corpus callosum**. Typical features of frontal lobe epilepsy are listed in **Table 9**. Electrical activity in one part of the brain quickly spreads to the other side. The frontal lobe seizures are shorter in duration. These tend to occur during the night. Patients typically have seizures during night time while sleeping. Patients may or may not experience an aura. Temporal lobe seizures

corpus callosum

A band of nerves that integrates the functions of the two halves of the brain.

Table 9   Features of Frontal Lobe Seizures
Brief (seconds to less than a minute)
Frequent
Tend to occur in the night
Complex behavior
Screaming
Patients return to baseline very quickly
EEG may be completely normal in between the seizures
EEG changes are hard to appreciate during seizures

are rather bland in onset. Frontal lobe seizures involve very complex motor phenomenon and bilateral body movements. These can be associated with loud vocalization such as screaming, humming, or expletives. These are very commonly confused with **nonepileptic seizures** or sleep disorders. These tend to last less than 1 minute. Patients snap out of it very quickly, as if nothing happened. But these can occur frequently and tend to cluster, and can cause disruption of sleep. Children with frontal lobe epilepsy have chaotic sleep patterns; some are afraid to sleep at night, fearing seizures during sleep. Patients feel tired, fatigued, and sleepy during the day. They might experience headaches during the daytime because of lack of proper sleep and might have postictal headaches. In between the seizures, it is so hard to find any epilepsy brain waves on their EEGs. This is in contrast to patients with temporal lobe epilepsy, in which EEGs show frequent epilepsy spikes.

Temporal lobe epilepsy is the most common partial epilepsy. Patients with temporal lobe epilepsy can have one of the following three kinds of seizures:

1. Simple partial seizure
2. Complex partial seizure
3. Tonic-clonic seizure

Complex partial seizures cause impairment of consciousness. This impairment can vary from being very subtle and inconspicuous to a complete state of confusion and disorientation. The complex partial seizure may start as a simple partial seizure. **Simple partial seizure** is also called **aura**. The presence of auras strongly suggests partial epilepsy unless proven otherwise. Patients with generalized epilepsies typically do not get auras.

nonepileptic seizures (NES)

Abnormal behavior that can resemble a seizure but is not the result of excitation of cortical neurons.

temporal lobe epilepsy

Epilepsy in which the seizures originate in the temporal lobe of the brain. The seizures are usually complex partial seizures.

simple partial seizure

A partial seizure in which the person remains fully conscious but experiences unusual sensations such as strange tastes or smells, feelings of fear or déjà vu, or involuntary twitching of limbs.

aura

Warning before a seizure that the patients can recall. It is also called simple partial seizure.

Some patients report only big seizures to their physicians without realizing that even these auras are seizures. Simple partial seizures have no impairment in the level of consciousness. Different common auras, symptoms during the seizure, and after effects of seizures, are listed in **Table 10**. The seizures arising from the temporal lobe can spread to other areas of the brain because of rich connections to the other parts of the brain. This spread can cause a tonic-clonic or a grand mal seizure. This phenomenon of a partial seizure starting as a simple partial seizure (aura), then evolving into a complex partial seizure and then into a tonic-clonic seizure or convulsive phase is called **secondary generalization**. However, it may start as a simple partial seizure, but patients may go into a state of altered consciousness and may not have any warning. In such cases, patients have no recollection of their auras and do not recall what happened to them during the seizure. It may be even harder for them to keep a count of their seizures unless the seizures are witnessed or the patient suffers from physical injuries or wakes up with sore muscles, a bitten tongue, a bad headache, and/or changed surroundings around them.

secondary generalization
A partial seizure starts from a focus and then spreads within the brain causing convulsive seizures. This process is called secondary generalization.

Temporal lobe epilepsy can be medial or lateral. The medial part of the brain lies on the inner part of the brain, and the lateral part lies on the outer surface of the temporal lobe. The medial part has an important structure called the hippocampus, which is important for memory, spatial navigation, and learning. It is a seahorse shaped structure, which is affected in Alzheimer's disease as well. Children with febrile seizures can later develop medial temporal lobe epilepsy after a dormant period. These children may develop a medial temporal sclerosis or **hippocampal atrophy (Figure 3)**, which is a classic finding on an MRI. The cells in this part of the

hippocampal atrophy
Shrinkage or volume loss in the hippocampus.

Table 10 Common Symptoms Experienced by Patients Before, During, and After Seizures

Sensory/Thought	Emotional	Physical
Early Seizure Symptoms (Aura) • Smell • Sound • Taste • Visual loss or blurring • Déjà vu • Jamais vu • Racing thoughts • Forced thoughts • Depersonalization • Derealization • Abdominal sensations • Strange, hard to describe sensations • Tingling sensations	• Fear • Anxiety • Panic • Pleasant feeling	• Dizziness • Headache • Lightheadedness • Nausea • Numbness
Seizure Symptoms (Ictal) • Blackout • Confusion • Muffling of sounds • Electric shock sensation • Loss of consciousness • Smell • Spacing out • Out-of-body experience • Visual loss or blurring • Muffling of sounds/deafness	• Fear • Panic	• Staring • Chewing/swallowing movements • Grinding teeth • Smacking lips • Racing heart • Speaking difficulties • Breathing difficulties • Vocalization (making sounds) • Drooling • Fluttering eyelids • Tremors • Sweating • Eyes rolling up • Falling down • Inability to move • Stiffening • Incontinence (stools or urine) • Twitchings • Convulsions
After-Seizure Symptoms (Postical) • Memory loss • Writing difficulty	• Confusion • Depression • Fear • Frustration • Embarrassment • Psychosis	• Physical injuries • Difficulty talking • Sleeping • Exhaustion/tiredness • Headache • Nausea/vomiting • Thirst • Urge to urinate or defecate

Source: Reproduced from Singh A. 2006. *100 Questions and Answers About Epilepsy.* Sudbury, Massachusetts: Jones and Bartlett Publishers, LLC.

brain are very susceptible to complete lack of oxygen (anoxia) or partial lack of oxygen (hypoxia). The architecture of the cells of the temporal lobe changes over months to years (dormant period) after the initial insult and facilitates perpetuation of electrical microcircuits, transforming these into full-blown seizures.

The nature of this insult can vary and can be genetic or acquired. Acquired insults include febrile seizures, head trauma, low- or high-grade brain tumors, abnormal morphology of the cortex, encephalitis, or meningitis. Herpes virus has a predilection to involve temporal lobes.

17. What is status epilepticus?

Status epilepticus (SE) is a neurological emergency. It is defined as seizure activity continuously lasting at least 5 minutes. It is either continuous or two or more discrete seizures between which the patient does not return to baseline. That means that there is no recovery of consciousness, or it is incomplete. A previous definition of SE emphasized duration as 30 minutes. However, the current belief is to treat seizures aggressively if seizures do not stop on their own within 5 minutes. The status can be convulsive or nonconvulsive. Convulsive status is easy to recognize, but nonconvulsive status can be very hard to recognize and has serious implications. Morbidity and mortality is highest in newborns and young infants less than 6 months of age. **Table 11** sheds light on some of the medical complications of status epilepticus.

Nonconvulsive status can present with confused state or altered mental state. Based on the seizure type, the sta-

Table 11 Complications of Status Epilepticus
Irregularities in the heart rate: increase or decrease
Heart failure
Alterations in the breathing pattern
Blood pressure fluctuations
Breakdown of muscles (with continuous convulsions)
Lack of oxygen to brain
Dehydration
Fever
Brain swelling
Acute kidney failure
Fluids in the lungs

tus is also referred to by different names. **Table 12** refers to a different kind of status. Status treatment is based on ensuring patient airway, breathing, and adequate circulation. The physician makes sure that there is an intravenous access so that drugs can be infused. The drugs could be given intramuscularly in the beginning, if there is no access to an intravenous route. SE can occur at any

Table 12 Types of Status Epilepticus
Convulsive: Partial or generalized
Tonic-clonic status
Myoclonic status
Absence status
Clonic status
Tonic status (seen in children with Lennox-Gastaut syndrome)
Epilepsia partialis continua
Partial status epilepticus
Nonconvulsive: Partial or generalized
Absence status
Epilepsia partialis continua (seen with brain tumors and Rasmussen's encephalitis)
Electrical status epilepticus during sleep (ESES)
Special circumstances
Neonatal: Electrical seizures with persistence of abnormal state
Febrile status
Status with acute stroke
Status in HIV patients

age. The first seizure can present with SE in 55–70% of children. The highest incidence of SE is seen in children less than 1 year old. This age group has the highest incidence of recurrence, at close to 11%. Over 50% of SE in children occurs in children less than 3 years old. About 30% of children with SE develop epilepsy later. Children with febrile SE carry a higher risk of recurrence. The risk of an unprovoked seizure after SE over a 10-year period is close to 40%.

SE can be a consequence of some kind of brain insult. Some of the common causes are shown in **Table 13**.

18. My child is exhibiting bizarre behavior since I separated from my husband. He had one of his episodes in his pediatrician's office. I was told that these could be nonepileptic seizures. What are nonepileptic seizures?

Nonepileptic seizures (NES) are also called psychogenic seizures. This is considered a **somatoform disorder**, meaning subconscious production of symptoms due to psychological overflow. This is also referred as **conversion disorder**. This disorder is not so well studied in children. About 20–50% of the epilepsy monitoring admissions turn out to be nonepileptic seizures. About 4–20% of children admitted for video EEG are diagnosed with NES. Limited data on NES in children

somatoform disorder

A disorder characterized by a lot of physical complaints by the patient. These complaints sound like medical illnesses but cannot fit into a typical disease pattern.

conversion disorder

A psychological condition in which physical symptoms arise from the stress at a subconscious level.

Table 13 Common Causes of Status Epilepticus	
• Hypoxia	• Ischemia
• Meningitis	• Encephalitis
• Acute stroke	• Brain tumors
• Head trauma	• Abrupt withdrawal of antiepileptics
• Electrolytes imbalance	• Metabolic disorders

indicate no major sex predilection in children less than 13 years of age. In adolescence, there is a female predominance. NES are more common in children with partial epilepsy. Several other disorders may be associated with NES, such as anxiety, depression, tension or migraine headaches, or attention-hyperactivity disorders. About 15–20% of adult epilepsy patients have NES. Family members and healthcare workers may have difficulty differentiating nonepileptic seizures from epileptic seizures.

The diagnosis of nonepileptic seizures should be suspected when seizures are frequent despite being treated with appropriate medications and optimal dosages. About 20% of SE patients are found to have pseudo status. The word *pseudo* means false. The clinical features may vary. Children may lie motionless without much response. Or they could display very dramatic motor behavior with thrashing and flailing and irregular, erratic movements. Movements during epileptic seizures are synchronous. Nonepileptic movements occur in an asynchronous manner. Body rocking movements, crying, abrupt periods of responsiveness and unresponsiveness and pelvic thrusting movements are common. These tend to last longer than typical epileptic seizures. Epileptic seizures tend to last 2–3 minutes, while nonepileptic seizures can last up to 10–15 minutes. Nonepileptic seizures are misdiagnosed as epileptic seizures by the family members. On the other hand, frontal lobe seizures have been misdiagnosed as NES. In children and adolescents, these have to be differentiated from sleep disorders or shuddering attacks. Epileptic seizures are usually characterized by stereotyped behavior if there is only one focus. The behavior in NES can vary; the patients have uncoordinated movements, which start and stop and may alter by suggestion. Intermittent shaking, screaming, tensing up of facial muscles, stiffening of legs alternately, contraction of pelvic muscles, and arching movements of the back are common in children with NES. The EEG remains normal during NES. Once the diagnosis is confirmed, the patient should be weaned off of antiepileptics.

NES tend to be provoked by emotional stress and are seen more commonly in patients with previous psychiatric diagnoses, depression, and personality disorders. These patients may have a history of physical or sexual abuse. The Patel group from Indiana has reported stereotyped behavior in some children with NES, including subtle motor movements seen with younger children and aggressive, flailing movements in older children. Sometimes, the behavior is hard to distinguish from partial seizures. To make things more complicated, some patients may have partial seizures with coexisting NES. The detailed description of events and their duration can help your physician to tease out the difference between the two. **Table 14** shows some of the important differences between the epileptic and nonepileptic seizures. It is important to distinguish between the two because the treatment options for NES and epileptic seizures are different. Children and adolescents with NES continue to have events for a longer time than adults who have NES. Treatment is intensive psychotherapy and antidepressants or antianxiety drugs. Neuropsychiatric assessment should be done to understand the psychosocial stressors in the child's life. Prognosis is good if the diagnosis is accepted in a positive manner and diligent follow-up with a psychiatrist and psychotherapist is pursued.

Table 14 Differential Diagnosis of Epileptic and Nonepileptic Seizures

Characteristics	Epileptic seizures	Nonepileptic seizures
Onset	Abrupt	Gradual
Timing of seizures	Can occur any time	Tend to occur in the presence of witnesses
Duration	Typically 2–3 minutes	5 minutes or longer
Motor activity	Synchronous	Motor movements start and stop and are asynchronous
Eyes	Open	Closed
Breathing	Forced, regular, and deep	Slow, shallow, and irregular
Body movements	Head and body side-to-side	No side-to-side movements
Confusion after seizure	Usually present	Usually absent
Changes in seizure activity	No alteration with suggestion	Alteration with suggestion
Pelvic thrusting	Absent	Present
EEG	Abnormal	No changes

19. My daughter's seizures are not responding to any treatment. She is getting weaker on the left side where she has constant jerking movements. She was suspected to have Rasmussen's encephalitis. Can you explain?

It is a very tough call. Your daughter's repeat MRI of the brain shows shrinkage of the right side of the brain. This clinical presentation is suspicious of what we call **Rasmussen's encephalitis**. It is believed to be the result of autoimmune inflammation of the brain, which primarily involves one side of the brain. This disease could start locally but then spread to the adjacent areas on the same side. Rasmussen's encephalitis is a disease of childhood and adolescence. There are rapidly progressive forms evolving over weeks to months and other forms with a more indolent clinical course. As you may know, the right side of the brain controls the left side of the

Rasmussen's encephalitis

An autoimmune disease characterized by intractable seizures as a result of inflammation of the brain. Usually one hemisphere of the brain is spared.

body. So, in your daughter's case, I suspect that the right side of the brain is affected.

Children typically present with seizures. Seizures are partial in nature with or without loss of consciousness. Simple partial seizures (no alteration in the level of consciousness) can be completely resistant to medication therapy. This is referred as **epilepsia partialis continua**. The way the seizures present depends on the area of the brain that is involved. If motor areas are affected, jerking movements are noted during seizures. Involvement of the language areas affects expression or comprehension of the speech. Focal inflammation ultimately spreads to contiguous areas, and simple partial seizures may become complex partial (with altered level of consciousness) or generalized. The parts of the brain under constant irritation are unable to perform their normal functions. That explains the weakness your child has been experiencing. A brain MRI done a few weeks to months later may reveal shrinkage of the affected side of the brain. Patients have **glutamate** receptor antibodies (Glu R3) in their blood. These antibodies bind to the brain cells and can be detected in the spinal fluid. A spinal tap excludes other common infections—viral or bacterial. A brain biopsy can confirm the diagnosis. Surgical **resection** of the involved hemisphere (**hemispherectomy**; see Question 93) can help the seizures if the diagnosis of Rasmussen's is confirmed based on the following:

- Clinical presentation
- Atrophy of the brain on the serial MRI
- Glu R3 antibodies
- Brain biopsy suggestive of Rasmussen's encephalitis.

Classification of Seizures

epilepsia partialis continua

Continuous twitching of one group of muscles at regular intervals lasting for hours or months. Movements occur on one side of the body and can continue throughout sleep.

glutamate

An excitatory neurotransmitter.

resection

Excision of a portion or all of an organ or other structure.

hemispherectomy

Removal of most areas of one side of the brain (usually diseased part of the brain); also involves disconnection between the two hemispheres. This is done in patients with uncontrolled seizures.

20. What is tuberous sclerosis?

Tuberous sclerosis (TS) is a neurological disorder that affects multiple organ systems. It is a neurological disease that is commonly diagnosed between 2 and 5 years of age. Some cases may be recognized prior to birth or in utero. Some cases are not appropriately diagnosed as late as adolescence. The disorder often involves the brain, heart, kidneys, eyes, skin, and nails. The skin condition is commonly confused with acne. Some patients have abnormal outgrowths in the fingernails and toenails. A brain MRI may show numerous collections of abnormal neurons, clumped as **tubers** (potatoes) as indicated by arrows in **Figure 6**. A tuber is a benign tumor of the brain that involves the cerebral cortex. Abnormal collections of disorganized nerve cells give rise to seizures.

tuber

Abnormal, disorganized large neuron cell in the cortex; seen in tuberous sclerosis.

A second type of brain lesion is seen in patients with tuberous sclerosis near the fluid spaces called ventricles. These lesions abut the lining of the ventricles and are

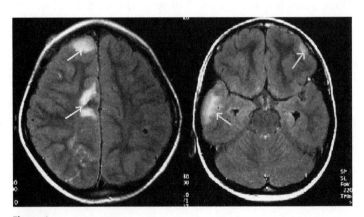

Figure 6
MRI of the brain with multiple tubers as indicated by arrows. *Source:* Reproduced from Singh A. 2006. *100 Questions and Answers About Epilepsy.* Sudbury, Massachusetts: Jones and Bartlett Publishers, LLC.

called **subependymal nodules**. These usually do not grow and do not need to be surgically removed.

The third type of brain lesion is called **subependymal giant cell astrocytoma**, abbreviated as **SEGA**. As these tumors grow, they can obstruct the cerebrospinal fluid flow and result in obstructive **hydrocephalus** (hydro = water; cephalus = brain). The patients may suddenly present with acute neurologic emergency. They may experience severe headache, nausea, vomiting, and visual disturbances. This requires the placement of a shunt in the brain for drainage of the fluid in the brain.

Abnormal tissue proliferation can occur in other organs such as the heart, kidneys, eyes, and lungs. The child needs an ultrasound of the heart and kidneys to look for these tumors. About 50% of the patients have heart tumors. These are called **cardiac rhabdomyomas** and can be multiple or single. These might be present at birth and do not appear later on in life, unlike kidney and lung tumors. In fact, they may disappear or decrease in size as the child grows. The functioning of the heart can be affected by the tumors. A child may develop problems with the pumping action of the heart or there can be rhythm problems. The **electrocardiogram**, echocardiogram, and Holter monitor (a 24-hour heart monitor to evaluate rhythm abnormalities) are common cardiac tests required for complete evaluation.

TS is recognized by myriad skin stigmata. The common skin manifestations associated with TS are as follows:

- Café-au-lait spots
- Adenoma sebaceum (facial angiomas)
- Shagreen patch

subependymal nodules

Nodules that are composed of calcified glia (supporting cells of the brain) and vascular elements that are found in the ventricles.

subependymal giant cell astrocytoma (SEGA)

Approximately 15% of the patients with tuberous sclerosis develop a midline tumor in the frontal areas of the brain that can cause obstruction to the flow of the cerebrospinal fluid.

hydrocephalus

An enlargement of the head caused by an abnormal buildup of cerebrospinal fluid.

cardiac rhabdomyomas

Tumors of the heart commonly associated with tuberous sclerosis.

electrocardiogram (EKG)

A recording that shows the electrical activity of the heart over time.

Classification of Seizures

Koenen tumors

Skin growths seen around toe and finger nails in patients with tuberous sclerosis.

café-au-lait spots

Light brown to dark brown skin lesions with smooth or irregular borders.

adenoma sebaceum

A skin condition seen in tuberous sclerosis. It affects face and nose, and can look like acne.

shagreen patch

Areas of thick leathery skin that are usually found on the lower back or nape of the neck.

periungual fibromas

Fibrous growths of the toe and finger nails as seen in tuberous sclerosis.

- Periungual fibromas (**Koenen tumors**)
- Forehead plaque
- Confetti lesions

Patients with TS can have leaf-shaped, hypopigmented (light color or whitish) spots on the skin. Melanin normally pigments the normal skin. Lightly colored areas are deficient in melanin and are called **café-au-lait spots**. Café-au-lait spots are better visualized with a Wood's lamp. A Wood's lamp transmits ultraviolet light with a filter that only passes light with a certain wavelength. Café-au-lait spots are different from another common condition called vitiligo. Vitiligo is seen early on in life or during infancy. Some normal newborns may have whitish spots without any neurological disease. However, a possibility of tuberous sclerosis should be considered in a child with more than three café-au-lait spots.

Another common skin condition is called **adenoma sebaceum**. This can be confused with acne. It is present in about 50% of the TS patients. These may be present as early 2–3 years of age and tend to increase in size as the child grows old. These lesions affect the skin around the nose, cheeks, or chin.

A **shagreen patch** is found in the back; it is usually a rough, textured, darkly pigmented area, which is raised from the skin surface. **Periungual fibromas** are more commonly seen on toes than fingers. These are like pinkish skin growths near the toe and fingernail folds.

TS can affect the child's eyes. The colored part of the eyes, called the iris, can have the whitish spots just like skin café-au-lait spots. The back of the eye, called the retina, can have tumor-like growths called **retinal hemartomas** and mulberry lesions.

About 50–65% of patients have involvement of their kidneys. Kidneys can harbor benign renal cysts on both sides, malignant tumors called **angiomyolipomas**, or renal cell carcinomas. These can enlarge or bleed into the kidney. Angiomyolipomas can develop anytime from childhood into adulthood. Malignant tumors of the kidney may require removal of part or all of the kidney. **Rapamycin** is the drug that shows activity against kidney tumors in TS. The renal angiomyolipomas shrink significantly in some patients after the use of rapamycin, obviating the need for surgery. Unfortunately, rapamycin does not cross the blood–brain-barrier. Lung tumors are also seen in patients with TS, but these are more common in adult women than men.

The association of tuberous sclerosis with neurological and nonneurological disorders is summarized in **Table 15**.

There is a **forme fruste** form of TS, where we find isolated cortical tubers on CAT scan or MRI of the brain without other stigmata of disease. The age of onset of seizures can be delayed as late as adulthood. Patients do not have positive family history.

retinal hemartomas
Abnormal growths in the retina.

angiomyolipomas
A tumor of fat and muscle tissue that is usually found in the kidney. These are common in patients with tuberous sclerosis and are considered benign tumors but may bleed requiring removal of kidneys.

rapamycin
An antibiotic that blocks a protein involved in cell division. This drug is also called *sirolimus*. It has been used to prevent the rejection of organ or bone marrow transplants by the body.

forme fruste
A form of tuberous sclerosis where tubers are found in the brain without involvement of other organs such as skin, heart, eyes, or kidneys.

Table 15 Common Associations with Tuberous Sclerosis in Percentages	
Epilepsy	80–90%
Skin lesions	70–80%
Mental retardation	60–70%
Kidney disease	50–65%
Cardiac disease	50–60%
Autism	16–58%

Classification of Seizures

PART THREE

Diagnostic Testing

What is an electroencephalogram?

What is the difference between a CAT scan and
an MRI of the brain? Which one is better?

Would my child require sedation for the tests?
What sedation would you use?

More ...

An electroen-cephalogram (EEG) meas-ures the electri-cal activity of the brain.

21. What is an electroencephalogram?

An electroencephalogram (EEG) measures the electrical activity of the brain. The brain cells communicate with each other by producing minor electrical impulses. It is an indirect way of knowing how the brain is functioning by measuring the electrical rhythm of the brain. The brain has different rhythms in different regions and different states. The rhythm may be different when your child is relaxed compared to when he or she is tense. The doctor sees different rhythms when the patient is sleeping than when he or she is awake. The EEG recording displays a mixture of different frequencies (number of waves in 1 second). The technician measures the patient's head and places electrodes on the scalp in multiple areas. **Figure 7** shows scalp electrodes used to record brain waves. Scalp electrodes are placed using a special technique. The technique uses the distance between bony landmarks on the scalp and generates lines. These lines intersect at intervals of 10% or 20% of

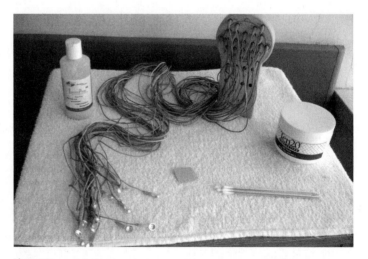

Figure 7
Scalp electrodes used to record EEG tracings. *Source:* Reproduced from Singh A. 2006. *100 Questions and Answers About Epilepsy.* Sudbury, Massachusetts: Jones and Bartlett Publishers, LLC.

their total length, thus it is called the **international 10–20 system**. These electrodes are glued to the scalp and left on until the EEG is finished. This glue is sticky, but the technician helps remove the glue once the test is complete. It is important that the child stays still during the procedure. EEG is very prone to what we call *artifacts*. There could be many artifacts. Practically any kind of movement could interfere with the quality of recording. If the child is using a pacifier, crying, or if a parent is patting the child's back to calm him or her, such an action would produce artifacts in the EEG. Eye movements, heartbeat, respiration, muscle activity and movement, chewing, swallowing, and sweating can cause artifacts.

If the child is uncooperative, then he or she might require sedation. Chloral hydrate is the most frequently employed sedative for this purpose. It is safe and effective. The sedative effect lasts long enough to apply electrodes and record the sleep EEG. The advantage of this agent is that it does not affect the EEG rhythms, while other sedatives can alter the background EEG rhythms, making it harder for interpretation. The need for sedation can be avoided by full preparation of parents and the child and creating a child-friendly environment before the study. Sometimes children are better off in a parent's lap than lying on the stretcher or bed. Children may be distracted by showing them some videos or cartoon films while electrodes are being placed or the EEG is being recorded. **Figure 8** represents a normal EEG recording in an awake, relaxed, and cooperative child.

Three special procedures are done during an EEG. The patient is encouraged to go to sleep; this is called **sleep induction**. In some patients, only sleep shows abnormalities in the EEG. Therefore, the EEG technician

international 10-20 system

A system where the head is measured between the two bony landmarks (reference points) and then the electrodes are placed at a certain distance. The gap between the 2 electrodes is 10% or 20% of the total length between the 2 reference points.

sleep induction
Inducing sleep.

Diagnostic Testing

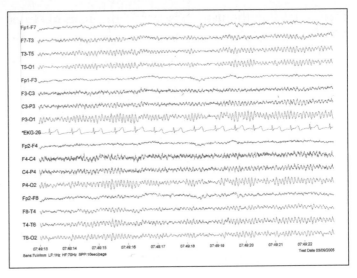

Figure 8
Normal EEG tracings in an awake and relaxed child. *Source:* Reproduced from Singh A. 2006. *100 Questions and Answers About Epilepsy.* Sudbury, Massachusetts: Jones and Bartlett Publishers, LLC.

hyperventilation
Rapid, deep breathing.

photic stimulation
Stimulation of the brain by flashing light or alternating patterns of light and dark.

activation procedures
Common procedures done while doing an EEG. Hyperventilation (deep breathing) and photic stimulation (strobe light stimulation) are the two commonly used activation procedures done during EEG recording.

always makes an attempt to acquire some sleep recording during the EEG. The other two procedures are called **hyperventilation** and **photic stimulation**. These are called **activation procedures**, as they may activate the abnormal patterns in the EEG.

Hyperventilation is nothing but the deep breathing exercise. This is performed for 3–5 minutes. In children, this deep breathing produces slowing of waves, if the effort is good. This slowing appears intermittently and soon after the deep breathing is started. In children, this slowing is seen maximally in the back areas of the head. In contrast, adults or teenagers are found to have this slowing more in the frontal regions of the head. This normal response finishes within 1 minute after the hyperventilation is stopped. Normal children may have brief lapses of awareness during hyperventilation; these lapses should not be misinterpreted as seizures.

Photic stimulation uses different frequencies of strobe light consisting of flashes of light.

Certain stages of sleep can activate abnormal epilepsy brain waves. Hyperventilation is known to exacerbate generalized epilepsies—particularly absence seizures. At least 30% of generalized epilepsies can be activated by strobe light stimulation (see Figure 5). On occasions, these activation procedures may provoke full-blown seizures. Photic stimulation and hyperventilation should be stopped if that is the case. Children with asthma and heart disease should not be subjected to hyperventilation.

A standard EEG is done for 40 minutes. Sometimes physicians may ask for a shorter or a longer study. Sleep-deprived EEG has a higher yield of picking up abnormality compared to a routine EEG. In a sleep-deprived EEG, you deprive your child of sleep the night before his or her EEG appointment. The chances are higher that your child would go to sleep when the test is done.

Epileptic seizures are stereotyped most of the time and show changes on the EEG. We see a change in clinical behavior associated with the EEG changes. On occasions, the clinical changes may not be obvious, but EEG indicates seizure-like activity. These are called **electrographic seizures**.

An **ambulatory electroencephalogram** monitoring allows prolonged EEG recording in the home setting. An ambulatory electroencephalogram is a less expensive alternative to inpatient monitoring and cuts health costs significantly by obviating the need for hospital admission. The length of monitoring can vary from 24 hours to 72 hours but can be extended for longer periods.

electrographic seizures

EEG pattern suggestive of seizures without clinical manifestations. Also called subclinical seizures.

ambulatory electroencephalogram

A portable type of EEG that allows the electrical activity of the brain to be recorded over a period of several hours or several days at home.

22. What is the difference between a CAT scan and an MRI of the brain? Which one is better?

Magnetic resonance imaging (MRI) of the brain is a frequently ordered test in patients with epilepsy. An MRI is a noninvasive procedure that gives a two-dimensional view of the brain without radiation exposure This technique is based on the magnetic fields generated from the hydrogen atoms in the body. The magnetic fields align the spinning of atoms in water molecules. A brain image is created as small amounts of energy are released when the atoms relax to their normal state. The computer analyzes these magnetic fields and generates pictures of the brain. The brain picture may or may not be able to determine the cause of epilepsy. That is why sometimes the MRI of the brain shows nothing abnormal even though the patient has epilepsy. The techniques we have are pretty sophisticated but still may not be enough to delineate the abnormalities at a microscopic or chemical-level to determine responsibility for abnormal excitation in the brain. Patients with epilepsy should have a special MRI of the brain. This is called the **MRI of the brain with seizure protocol**, where special attention is given to temporal lobes. **Figure 9** shows special MRI protocol used in patients with seizures showing shrinkage of the left hippocampus.

An MRI of the brain may show different abnormal features. Some common ones include stroke, previous brain injury due to head trauma, tumor (benign and malignant), infection, scar tissue, abnormal blood vessel, or abnormal pool of brain cells.

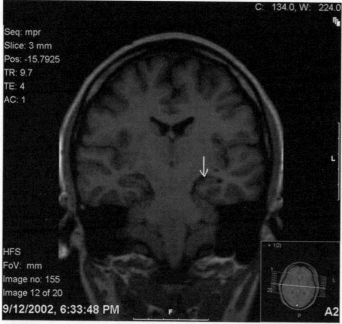

Seq: mpr
Slice: 3 mm
Pos: -15.7925
TR: 9.7
TE: 4
AC: 1

C: 134.0, W: 224.0

L

HFS
FoV: mm
Image no: 155
Image 12 of 20
9/12/2002, 6:33:48 PM

A2

Figure 9
MRI of the brain—seizure protocol showing left hippocampal shrinkage shown by an arrow. *Source:* Reproduced from Singh A. 2006. *100 Questions and Answers About Epilepsy.* Sudbury, Massachusetts: Jones and Bartlett Publishers, LLC.

A **computed axial tomography (CAT) scan** can also reveal traumatic brain injuries, hemorrhage, scar tissue, strokes, tumors, abnormal blood vessels, or shrinkage of the brain. **Figure 10** shows the CAT scan of a brain with collection of blood in the coverings of the brain called epidural hematoma. The use of CAT scans in the United States started in the early 1970s. The CAT scan exposes the patient to the risk of radiation, just like X-rays. The advantages of CAT scan include lower cost, easy availability in most places, and fast processing time. The CAT scan is a very reasonable alternative or an option when patients are uncooperative or claustrophobic. MRI is better than a CAT scan because it provides

computerized axial tomography (CAT) scan

A brain scan showing anatomy of the brain using X-rays.

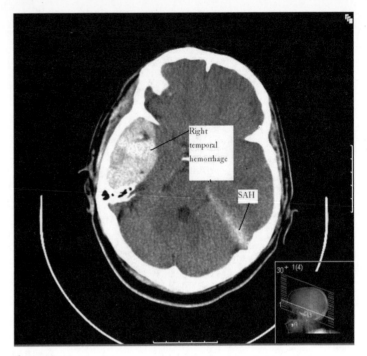

Figure 10
CAT scan of the brain in a patient with head trauma showing right temporal hemorrhage and left subarachnoid hemorrhage (SAH).

images with better resolution of the soft tissues. A CAT scan is not so good in discriminating the gray and white matter. The lower part of the brain called the *brain stem* may not be adequately visualized on the CAT scan because of streak artifacts from the bones. A CAT scan is helpful if there is blood or calcium in the brain. MRI is a better way of looking at soft tissues. MRI technique is more expensive and may not be available at all centers. It may be hard for the parents to cover the cost of the MRI if their child does not have insurance. MRI takes a longer time to obtain images compared to a CAT scan. CAT scanning is more readily available in the emergency rooms; MRI is rarely available in emergency settings. There are no risks involved with the MRI except it may be contraindicated in certain situations. Presence

pacemaker

A small device that is implanted under the skin of the chest or abdomen to control heart rhythms.

of **pacemakers**, **metallic heart valves**, bullet fragments, metallic plates, and **internal defibrillator devices** are some of the absolute contraindications to MRI. Some MRI centers can do MRI on patients with a **vagal nerve stimulator (VNS)**, but ask patients to have it turned off before the MRI. Children with orthodontic braces or surgical metallic hardware in their body, such as plates, screws, or pins, do not pose any risk to obtain an MRI. MRI-compatible clips used to treat aneurysms (dilatation or outpouchings of the brain vessels) pose no extra risk either.

When MRI is contraindicated, a CAT scan remains a very reasonable option. The MRI cannot be obtained in patients who are intubated or connected to an artificial lung-heart machine or in a very sick child. MRI of the brain may not be necessary in patients with generalized epilepsies where the clinical picture indicates and the EEG data confirms the diagnosis of epilepsy.

Special MRI techniques such as **diffusion tensor imaging** can be extremely helpful in evaluating a patient with epilepsy under certain circumstances. Diffusion tensor imaging has the ability to detect areas of the brain that have restriction of the normal flow of water, possibly the **seizure focus**.

23. Would my child require sedation for the tests? What sedation would you use?

For a quality MRI, the child should lie still in the MRI machine for 20–40 minutes. It can be challenging for infants, toddlers, or even older children. Therefore, they require sedation so that they can remain motionless during the test. Older kids should be given a trial without

---

Diagnostic Testing

metallic heart valve

An artificial heart valve made of metal that is used in patients when natural valves of the heart are diseased and are malfunctioning. This may require open-heart surgery.

internal defibrillator device

Device that delivers small electrical energy to the affected heart. This device terminates the irregular heart beat and reestablishes the normal regular heart rhythm.

vagal nerve stimulator (VNS)

A small generator implanted in a person's chest. The generator stimulates the vagus nerve that may prevent the abnormal brain activity that gives rise to a seizure.

diffusion tensor imaging (DTI)

Measures the movement of water in the brain and detects areas where the normal flow of water is disrupted. A disrupted flow of water indicates where there could be an underlying abnormality.

seizure focus

Place where the seizure is originating; if there are multiple sources, they are called seizure foci.

sedation, as they may cooperate for the test. Lorazepam (Ativan) or diazepam can be given to children. Chloral hydrate, diazepam, thiopental, midazolam, or propofol can be used for sedation in children undergoing an MRI or CAT scan. Sometimes, pediatric anesthesia is required to obtain a quality MRI without motion artifacts, especially in children who are very young, mentally handicapped, or have neuropsychiatric issues. Anesthesia can be administered by giving intravenous anesthetics, or your child would breathe through a facial mask. The anesthesiologist monitors the blood pressure, pulse, respiration, and level of anesthesia throughout. The child wakes up very soon in the MRI area if everything goes well.

24. What is a video EEG? What information does it provide?

Video EEG is a long, continuous monitoring of brain waves (electroencephalogram) done both during sleep and wakefulness. When the doctor suspects irregular heartbeat or heart problems, the internist orders an electrocardiogram, which is a recording of the heartbeat. The brain exhibits different rhythms during different states of mind such as wakefulness, alertness, relaxation, or light or deep sleep. This test provides valuable information to the neurologist or epileptologist treating patients with seizures. This is an inpatient test in which your child is admitted to the hospital. Metallic electrodes are placed on your child's head and left on during the monitoring. Your child cannot take a shower or get her hair wet. It could be a short test for 24–48 hours, where your physician wants to confirm the diagnosis or try to determine what kind of epilepsy she has. The activation procedures such as deep breathing exercise and

A video EEG provides valuable information to the neurologist or epileptologist treating patients with seizures.

strobe light stimulation may be performed during the stay to provoke seizures. These are called hyperventilation and photic stimulation, respectively. Older children are asked to stay up until late in the night. Sleep deprivation, hyperventilation, and photic stimulation are some of the means to provoke seizures. The duration of the study varies from patient to patient. Children admitted for presurgical evaluation are required to stay longer. The average length of study is from 5 to 7 days. The length of stay in these patients varies depending on how quickly seizures are captured. This could be very anxiety provoking for the parents, but it is good to bear in mind that your child is in a safe environment where medical staff is well versed with the first-aid care your child may require. Most of the seizures are self-limiting and stop on their own.

You can also take a video of the seizures at home. This can help your physician to understand the nature of episodes. For presurgical evaluation, the aim is to capture 2–3 seizures in the hospital. On an average, this may require staying in the epilepsy unit for 5–7 days. The length of stay depends upon how quickly your physician is able to acquire the needed information. It can last longer when it is crucial to capture seizures and epilepsy surgery is contemplated.

25. What are epilepsy monitoring units?

An **epilepsy monitoring unit (EMU)** is a specially designed unit where patients get admitted for video EEG testing. It helps your physician to understand the kind of seizures your child has. A normal test does not refute or support the diagnosis of epilepsy. Patients are admitted for seizure characterization. An epileptologist

epilepsy monitoring unit (EMU)

A specialized unit where continuous EEG is done; this test is called video EEG.

reads the EEG. This helps him or her answer the following questions:

- Does your child have epilepsy and if yes, what kind—partial or generalized?
- From what part of the brain does the seizure start?
- Do all seizures start from one focus? Or are there different foci?
- Is that one focus very narrow or widespread?
- If there are different foci, is there any predominant focus from which most of the seizures were captured?
- Is the child on the right kind of medication(s)?
- Does the child have subclinical seizures? Subclinical seizures refer to no change in clinical behavior to suspect seizures, although the EEG shows clear-cut seizures. The subclinical seizures can be short or long, frequent or infrequent.
- Does the child have a very active EEG? Can a very active EEG or subclinical seizures explain any learning or behavioral problems?
- As the medications are being adjusted in a safer setting, with the guidance of EEG, does the EEG indicate improvement or worsening with the new medication(s)?

26. Why does my child need a spinal tap? What additional information would it give that was not obtained from the EEG and MRI of the brain?

A spinal tap is also called a lumbar puncture. The physician takes some **cerebrospinal fluid (CSF)** from the lower back. This fluid circulates in the brain and the spinal cord, which are in communication with each

cerebrospinal fluid

Fluid that runs in the brain and spinal cord.

other. Using sterile techniques, the physician takes this fluid by placing a needle between the two lower lumbar vertebrae. This procedure is needed under special circumstances when the causes of seizures are not clear. In the neonatal period, this test is frequently done to rule out infection. When your doctor suspects any infection such as meningitis (infection of coverings of the brain, called *meninges*) or encephalitis (infection of the brain), the spinal tap should be done as soon as possible. Various viral and bacterial cultures can be done on the CSF. A spinal tap is also indicated when bleeding around the brain or a metabolic or mitochondrial disease is suspected. A pediatric neurologist may have to work with the geneticist and do special tests, looking for lactate, pyruvate, glucose, glycine, and amino acid concentrations in the CSF.

27. How often does my child need blood tests? What are you monitoring?

The basic electrolytes and blood counts along with liver function tests should be done before starting medications. I would like to get a baseline blood test to eliminate the possibility of previously unrecognized underlying liver or kidney problems.

Drug levels or antiepileptic levels are measured in the blood. Only a part of the drug enters the bloodstream. The drug exists in the body in two forms, free and bound to proteins—mainly albumin. The drug levels reflect the total concentration in the blood. **Table 16** shows the normal range of drug levels of commonly used antiepileptic drugs (AEDs). This includes both free and bound drugs. The free drug goes through the

Table 16	Potential Target Range of Blood Levels of Commonly Used Antiepileptics
AED	**Blood levels (mg/l)**
Carbamazepine (Tegretol)	4–12
Divalproex sodium (Depakote)	50–100
Ethosuximide (Zarontin)	40–100
Felbamate (Felbatol)	50–100
Gabapentin (Neurontin)	6–21
Lamotrigine (Lamictal)	5–18
Levetiracetam (Keppra)	10–40
Oxcarbazepine (Trileptal)	12–24
Phenobarbital	15–40
Phenytoin (Dilantin)	10–20
Pregabalin (Lyrica)	10–20
Topiramate (Topamax)	4–25
Zonisamide (Zonegran)	7–40

blood–brain barrier and exerts its actions on the brain. The free drug levels can be high when the albumin concentration is low and the drug has no albumin to which it can bind. The albumin concentrations are low in neonates, in patients with liver and kidney disease, or during pregnancy. Under such circumstances, free levels are measured as well. Free levels can be checked in the blood or saliva.

The need to check the blood levels of antiepileptics and monitor blood counts varies from patient to patient. There is no hard and fast rule about the frequency at which blood tests should be done. If your child is doing well (no seizures and no side effects), then there is no need to do frequent blood tests. However, if there was an abnormal lab report in the past, the blood tests may be required on a regular basis to ensure that the drug can be continued safely. **Table 17** lists some special circumstances when blood monitoring is recommended. If there are frequent seizures or side effects, then blood levels give a rough idea to your child's physician. For example, some children manifest seizures if the level of

Table 17	Indications for Monitoring of Antiepileptic Drug Levels

To ensure that the patient is taking medications
Patients with signs or symptoms of drug toxicity
To check for drug-to-drug interactions in patients taking multiple
  medications
Patients with underlying kidney disease
Patients with underlying liver disease
Patients with low albumin concentration
Patients who are pregnant

the drug in their blood falls below a certain range. Physicians go over the side effects of medications at great length. If you think your child is experiencing any side effects, then the blood levels may be required.

Most of the drugs pass through the liver, get absorbed by the intestine, and then are excreted in the urine and stool. There are few exceptions, such as levetiracetam and gabapentin, which do not get metabolized by the liver. Certain drugs, such as felbamate, require blood monitoring on a regular basis. When the drug is started, the blood counts need to be done every 2 weeks. Patients on more than two or three AEDs require blood tests more frequently. There could be drug-to-drug interactions when two or three drugs are being used to treat epilepsy. AEDs can cause mild elevation in the liver enzymes. The elevation in the liver enzymes becomes significant if it is more than three times higher than the baseline. Other alternatives should be considered under such circumstances.

28. What is a neuropsychological evaluation?

A neuropsychological evaluation involves the assessment of cognitive functions that may be affected by various neurologic conditions. The information gained from the evaluation will help your child's neurologist with treatment planning, and it may help the school system gain a better understanding of your child and what types of educational interventions will benefit him or her. The testing is noninvasive in nature and can be completed as either an outpatient or as an inpatient.

The evaluation of children and adolescents involves several components. These include a review of records, parent interview, parental completion of questionnaires rating the child's behavior, cognitive function, and academic abilities, as well as a formal one-to-one testing of the child. The **neuropsychologist** may also wish to review school records, the child's individualized education plan (if he or she has one), or have the child's teacher complete various forms as well.

neuropsychologist

Physician who specializes in the relationship between the brain and how individuals think and behave.

A neuropsychological evaluation can take several hours, depending on several factors, including the age of the child and the child's abilities. Neuropsychological evaluations can be performed on children at any age, but the nature of the evaluation changes as the children age and their cognitive functions become more differentiated and mature. In very young children, the evaluation may involve more in the way of a structured parent interview and observation of the child, whereas in older children, testing is lengthier and more detailed, involving more one-to-one testing of the child. Children who are delayed from a cognitive perspective often require less formal testing, as they cannot tolerate lengthy sessions.

The information gained from a neuropsychological evaluation generally includes a measure of the child's level of general intellectual functioning (e.g., IQ), attention and concentration abilities, memory, language skills, visual spatial skills, and motor skills. A formal evaluation of mood and behavior is also commonly conducted, as well as an evaluation of academic skills (e.g., reading, writing, spelling, and mathematics) depending on the needs of the child and the specific referral question. These test procedures are not invasive in nature, and many seem like games to children. Children often find the tests enjoyable. Again, the actual length and timing of the evaluation must be tailored to the individual needs of the child. Often, the evaluation can be completed in a single visit (with breaks), but some children may require several testing sessions across a few days.

These test procedures are not invasive in nature, and many seem like games to children.

The main goal of the evaluation is to provide a picture of your child's strengths and weaknesses to optimize interventions and outcomes. The results of the evaluation may lead to specific recommendations such as investigating medications to improve cognitive function to be prescribed by the child's neurologist, interventions at school to minimize the impact of deficits, specific interventions to improve cognitive functions or academic abilities (e.g., reading interventions), and/or therapeutic plans to improve the child's mood and behavior at home or at school. Moreover, in the context of a comprehensive epilepsy evaluation, the neuropsychological evaluation is another method by which epileptologists lateralize and localize brain dysfunction prior to surgical interventions, as the pattern of cognitive strengths and weaknesses provides a picture of the integrity of the underlying neural systems. Your child may therefore benefit from a neuropsychological evaluation if he or she is to be undergoing surgical interventions for epilepsy. This often provides additional localization information prior to the surgery, but it also helps monitor outcomes over time. You may also wish to have a neuropsychological evaluation conducted if you suspect your child has problems with attention, memory, or language, or is having difficulty at school.

29. What is a magnetoencephalogram?

A **magnetoencephalogram** (**MEG**) identifies small magnetic fields generated by electrical currents produced by the firing of neurons. Magnetic fields can be very small and need sensors to amplify. MEG uses 248 channels instead of 32 channels used in scalp EEG, meaning a lot more electrodes are recording the brain's electric activity. It is a noninvasive test that measures intercellular currents of the neurons in the brain. These magnetic signals are measured by induction coils composed of loops of wire. The MEG assesses the function of the brain with more accuracy than the scalp EEG because of less distortion of the electrical signals. Events with time scales in the order of milliseconds can be localized. The sources of **epileptiform discharges** can be localized with millimeter precision. These sources can be superimposed on the MRI of the brain. This is called **magnetic source imaging**. Magnetic source imaging provides information about the structure and function of the brain. **Figure 11** depicts MEG dipoles on the coregistered MRI of a child's brain. Motor, sensory, language, memory, visual, and hearing areas can be demarcated on these magnetic source imaging images. Information provided by the MEG can provide useful information about the seizure foci and areas that need to be studied closely with the help of strips, a **grid**, and **depth electrodes**.

Young children may require sedation for MEG. EEG electrodes are glued to the child's head. Three small coils

---

magnetoencephalogram (MEG)

Noninvasive functional brain mapping that localizes electrical activity of the brain by measuring the associated magnetic fields emanating from the brain.

epileptiform discharge

Abnormal wave in an EEG in patients with epilepsy that indicates signs of excitation in the brain; also referred to as *epilepsy brain waves*.

magnetic source imaging (MSI)

Superimposition of MEG data on a magnetic resonance image (MRI).

grid

An array of multiple electrodes that is inserted after opening skull bone. It can cover a wider area of brain compared to strips.

depth electrodes

A specialized electrode made of polyurethane or other material that is inserted into the brain to help locate the seizure onset and has multiple contact points.

Diagnostic Testing

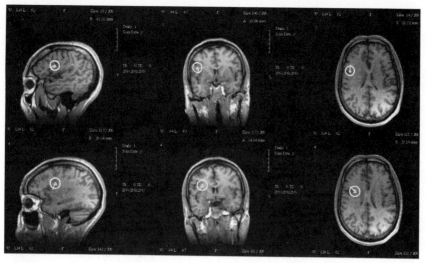

Figure 11
Magnetic source imaging localizes MEG epileptiform dipoles on the superimposed MRI.
Source: Reproduced from Singh A. 2006. *100 Questions and Answers About Epilepsy.*
Sudbury, Massachusetts: Jones and Bartlett Publishers, LLC.

get taped to the forehead, and two other coils are attached to earplugs. The MEG test takes between 1 hour and 2.5 hours. During this time, the child needs to remain as still as possible.

30. What is f-MRI?

A functional MRI is called an f-MRI. Advances in brain mapping with f-MRI have opened an important window into understanding how language is organized in the developing brain. Children with epilepsy, particularly those anticipating surgical intervention, may benefit from preoperative language localization with f-MRI, thus minimizing the risk of incurring new deficits.

An f-MRI is a blood-flow technique; it measures blood flow changes in brain regions. Activation of different brain regions increases their metabolic activity during a cognitive, sensory, or motor task. The f-MRI measures blood flow indirectly. During brain activation, blood flow increases and brings more oxygenated blood into the system. At the capillaries, however, the brain does not utilize the extra oxygen at nearly the rate at which it arrives, and as a consequence, a higher concentration of oxygenated blood slips over to the venous side. This lessens the magnetic field gradient and thus increases the MRI signals, which are strongly affected by inhomogeneous magnetic fields.

Functional MRI has a strong advantage over imaging like PET (see Question 31) in several respects relevant to pediatric imaging: it requires no ionizing radiation; there are no known risks; the studies may be repeated as often as necessary; and it is relatively easy to obtain sufficient data to achieve within-subject statistical significance. The latter advantage has particular relevance for pediatric imaging, in that we may expect a high degree of individual variability in language organization because of the increased neuroplasticity for language in children.

To obtain maps of brain activity, then, the researcher typically has the subject perform a series of activation and control tasks in blocks for a few minutes, during which images of the brain are continuously acquired, a volume every few seconds. It is important to record more observations per condition to differentiate between-condition differences from random variance in signal intensity. For instance, in a language task used in a laboratory, subjects rest for 30 seconds, name objects presented on a video screen every 5 seconds for 30 seconds, and repeat this for a total of three naming and four rest blocks, lasting 3 minutes and 30 seconds total. A volume of about seventeen slices is then acquired through the brain every 2.5 seconds, obtaining a sum of thirty-six images during naming and forty-eight at rest.

Unlike disruption mapping with direct cortical stimulation, which may show only those regions essential for language, f-MRI reveals any brain region involved in the task (less those showing activity in the control condition). Clinical application of f-MRI requires a thorough understanding of activations and control tasks, their replicability, and their consistency over time.

There are important potential clinical uses for functional MRI in mapping language functions in epileptic children; establishing hemispheric dominance and intrahemispheric localization of language sites prior to surgery and determining functional-neuroanatomical abnormalities in children with developmental language disorders are foremost among them. Before the advent of f-MRI, invasive procedures such as Wada testing (see Question 84) were used. However, studies now are showing concordant f-MRI and Wada testing results.

It was previously believed that language reorganization was not possible after the age of 7. So children who contracted epilepsy after the age of 7 and needed operative measures would do so at the cost of the deterioration of their language skills in some instances. The experimental use of f-MRI suggested that the right hemisphere was capable of assuming some basic language skills, even after the age of 7—though not at the level of sophistication that is possible in either early reorganization or in the normally functioning left hemisphere.

A disadvantage of f-MRI is that reducing head motion remains extremely difficult in very young children. To mitigate fear in young children, scanners are often designed like a spaceship. Precautions to reduce head motion may also include cushions, but while all of these tools *reduce* motion, they rarely *eliminate* it.

We can anticipate that future f-MRI research will establish normative data on language organization in the developing brain, which can serve as a basis of comparison for the benefit of children with epilepsy.

31. What is a PET scan?

Positron emission tomography (PET) is a diagnostic test that has been used in clinics on a regular basis since the 1990s. A radioactive material is injected intravenously into the arm 30 to 60 minutes before the patient is called for scanning. Scanning takes an additional 30 to 45 minutes. PET measures the metabolism of cells and thereby functioning of the cells. It is believed that the firing neurons during seizures are metabolically active. In between the seizures, the seizure focus has lower metabolism than the normal brain. PET and CT scanners can be combined so that the metabolic information is superimposed on the structure depicted on CT images of the brain. The most commonly used PET scans for epilepsy are **2-deoxy-2fluoro-D-glucose (FDG)**, **flumazenil**, and alpha-methyl-L-tryptophan (AMT). AMT-PET is particularly useful for children with tuberous sclerosis. This is a costly test. The price ranges from $900 to $4,000. This is an outpatient test. Patients are encouraged to drink water both before and

positron emission tomography (PET)

A brain scan that gives information about the function and the structure of the brain. It is a nuclear medicine test in which tissue function can be imaged. Damaged tissues have reduced metabolic activity; therefore, gamma radiation from these areas is reduced or absent.

2-deoxy-2fluoro-D-glucose (FDG)

A glucose analogue that is most commonly used in medical imaging such as PET. It is taken up by cells of organs with high glucose consumption and thereby reflects the distribution of glucose uptake.

flumazenil

An antidote used in the treatment of overdose of benzodiazepines.

after the test to flush the radioactive material. Patients should not eat for 4 hours before the scan. A radioactive substance is produced in a machine and is attached to a natural body compound such as glucose, water, or ammonia. Radioactivity exposure is very limited. Changes in metabolism are more widespread than the actual structural changes on the MRI or CT of the brain. PET is not as readily available as SPECT (see Question 32).

Patients are encouraged to drink water both before and after the test to flush the radioactive material.

32. What is a SPECT scan?

Single photon emission computerized tomography (SPECT) measures blood flow through different parts of the brain. Just like PET, a small dose of radioactive material is injected into the arm. This radioactive material emits particles called **gamma rays** that are detected by the scanner. It takes about 10 to 20 minutes before the radioactive material reaches the brain. The number of particles emitted is directly related to the blood flow in a region. The SPECT is a colorful display of different colors indicating different levels of blood flow **(Figure 12)**. There are two kinds of SPECT studies done in epilepsy patients—ictal and interictal. Ictal means seizure. A radioactive material is injected during a seizure. An interictal SPECT is the study done in between the seizures. During ictus there is an increased blood flow to the seizure focus. In between the seizures, there is decreased blood flow around seizure focus. SPECT is much more readily available and cheaper than the PET scan. There is less radiation exposure with SPECT compared to CAT scan. Patients are instructed to drink lots of fluids to flush out any tracer.

single photon emission computerized tomography (SPECT)

A type of brain scan that gives information about the function and structure of the brain.

gamma rays

Electromagnetic radiation emitted during radioactive decay that has an extremely short wavelength.

Diagnostic Testing

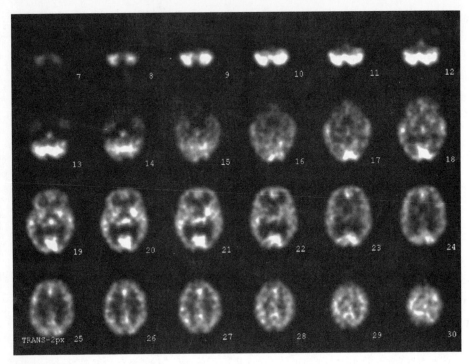

Figure 12
SPECT scan showing increased blood flow on the right side most evident in images 24–29 in the bottom two rows.
Source: Reproduced from Singh A. 2006. *100 Questions and Answers About Epilepsy*. Sudbury, Massachusetts: Jones and Bartlett Publishers, LLC.

PART FOUR

Treatment

Do all seizures need to be treated?

Does my child need to be treated after the first seizure?

How do I ensure the safety of my son during a seizure?

More ...

Provoked seizures do not need to be treated with antiepileptics.

33. Do all seizures need to be treated?

No, all seizures do not need to be treated with conventional therapy used for seizures. It is imperative to find out whether the seizures were provoked or unprovoked. *Provoked seizures do not need to be treated with antiepileptics.* These patients do not have underlying epilepsy. Electrolyte imbalance in the body, such as low or high glucose can cause seizures. Abnormal calcium, magnesium, and phosphate levels may lower the seizure threshold. During extreme stress (physical or mental), patients may have an isolated seizure. Hospital admissions to treat other medical complications may be confounded by such variables as hospital acquired infections or organ failures, and patients may experience one or more seizures during these extreme stressful periods. Surgeries under inhalational or intravenous anesthetics can be complicated by seizures. Prescribed, over-the-counter, or recreational drugs can lower the seizure threshold. Some antibiotics to treat infections, such as imipenem, or pain medications such as tramadol (Ultram), also lower seizure threshold. The list of pharmacological agents lowering seizure threshold is long. Common examples are narcotic pain medications, diet drugs, alcohol, brain stimulants, and some **antidepressants**. Severe sleep deprivation, strenuous exercise, and crash dieting (resulting in low glucose or any other electrolyte imbalance) can produce seizures. Children who have seizures due to the aforementioned causes do not need to be put on long-term treatment for epilepsy.

antidepressants

A group of drugs used to relieve symptoms of depression.

Once the cause of seizures is determined, the precipitating agent should be withdrawn or corrected. Correction of electrolytes and glucose imbalance, or stopping over-the-counter or prescribed medications, alcohol, or other recreational drugs would prevent seizures in the future if they are found to be the cause. Other medical conditions, such as heart rhythm irregularities, can cause seizures, and just the correction of irregular heartbeat with medical treatment or surgical intervention with a pacemaker can fix the underlying problem. In brief, treatment of the underlying cause can help prevent provoked seizures, and no conventional treatment for epilepsy is warranted. Febrile seizures do not need to be treated with antiepileptics unless they are prolonged, complicated, and frequent or have focal onsets.

More than two unprovoked seizures should be treated with antiepileptics. There is an 80–90% chance of recurrence of seizure after two unprovoked seizures **(Figure 13)**. One has to weigh risks and benefits of treating seizures and the side effects of medications. Strong seizures carry risk of physical injuries, such as lacerations, broken bones, dislocated shoulder, or other complications such as pneumonia, respiratory arrest, or sudden unexplained death. These risks are weighed against the side effects of medications. In partial

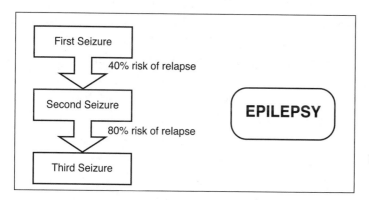

Figure 13
Risk of relapse after first or second unprovoked seizure without treatment.

epilepsy, if the MRI of the brain and EEGs have been normal and the patient is seizure free, then one attempt should be made to wean the patient off antiepileptics once the patient is seizure free for more than 2 years. Generally speaking, patients with generalized epilepsies can be successfully controlled with a low dose of antiepileptics, but they may need lifelong treatment.

34. Does my child need to be treated after the first seizure?

The first unprovoked seizure in a child always presents a dilemma. The decision to treat should take into consideration the risk factors for epilepsy, the child's overall development, a careful history, a physical, a thorough neurological assessment, lab data, brain MRI, and the EEG. The chances of recurrent seizure may range from 27% to 71%. Approximately 50% of recurrent seizures occur within the first 6 months of the first. More than 80% of seizures that have a recurrence do so within the next 2 years. We do not start the treatment after the first unprovoked seizure. The chances of recurrence are low if developmental milestones, neurological examination, MRI, and EEG are normal. The chance of recurrence is high when children have multiple risk factors. Children with previous neurological insult, age of onset more than 12 years, multiple seizure types, long duration of epilepsy, and persistent EEG abnormalities have a much higher recurrence risk of seizures. The benefits and risks of long-term treatment have to be kept in mind before starting treatment. If a child has more than two seizures, the possibility of seizure recurrence is more than 80% without treatment.

Children who are seizure free on medication for more than 2 years have a high probability of remaining in remission despite discontinuation. A longer seizure-free interval is associated with a lower recurrence risk; however, there is a potential risk of recurrence on withdrawal of medications. The chances of recurrence is higher under certain circumstances, such as abnormal EEG, remote brain insult, focal weakness after seizure, or complex partial seizure. Initiation of treatment after the first seizure is largely based on the test results and assessment of risk of relapse.

35. How do I ensure the safety of my son during a seizure?

You cannot do much to stop the seizure. Seizures stop on their own. Seizures can be mild or strong. If you catch your son in a complex partial seizure or a tonic-clonic seizure, you can certainly try the following steps to ensure his safety:

- Try to stay calm.
- Prevent falls.
- Prevent any other physical injuries; ensure that the surroundings are safe; guide him away from danger.
- Do not leave him unattended and in any dangerous situations.
- Loosen clothing.
- Turn him to the left to prevent aspiration.
- Do *not* put anything into his mouth!
- Do not restrain your son, as this may make him more apprehensive and confused.

If your son is having a seizure, do not put anything into his mouth!

- Ensure that he is breathing and the color of his skin looks good.
- During the convulsive phase, try to prevent injury of the head, arms, and legs caused by hitting the ground.

seizure alarm

A sensor technology that detects convulsions and triggers an alarm.

Seizure alarms are available that can alert the parents if their child has a seizure. A range of bed seizure alarms have been in production since 1996. Sensors are placed between the mattress and the base of the bed, and can detect the convulsive movements and the sounds made by your child during a grand mal seizure. The sensitivity of the sensors can be adjusted. Sleep-safe company specializes in anti-suffocation pillows. Hand or foot sensor units can be worn by the patient to distinguish movements of the body related to epileptic attacks from other movements. **Seizure dogs** are special dogs that have been trained to alert the family when a child has a seizure. These dogs can predict when people will have a seizure so that injuries during the seizures can be prevented.

seizure dogs

Trained dogs who act as helpers, protectors, and can even sense in advance when a person with epilepsy is going to have a seizure.

36. Should I call 911 if my daughter has a seizure?

You do not need to call 911 if your daughter has a seizure. Most of the seizures stop on their own. However, if this is her first seizure with or without fever, you should take her to the hospital for further workup. You should call 911 only if she does not snap out of it quickly and you are in doubt whether she is still "seizing" in the brain, has a cluster of seizures, or has prolonged seizures lasting more than 10–15 minutes. If any such event, she should be carefully watched in a hospital setting. Mostly children go to sleep after a prolonged seizure or may be confused or disoriented. It can be hard for you or even a physician to decide whether your daughter is in a postictal state or if she is still having seizures if she does not return to her baseline. Under such circumstances, you should definitely take no chances, and you should rush to the emergency room.

For a cluster of seizures or prolonged seizures, you should administer rectal **diazepam (Diastat)** at home. Whenever your daughter has prolonged seizures or back-to-back seizures, this is something you or a caregiver can do at home. This emergency treatment can be done at any place, not only in medical settings. If your daughter has frequent seizures, it is good to carry this drug with you if you are planning a vacation or she is attending a school or a summer program. It is one of the very valuable tools for families and caregivers of children with epilepsy. It is very easy to administer and comes with clear instructions. It aborts the prolonged seizure or cluster of seizures. We have more than 20 years experience with diazepam rectal gel worldwide. It comes in a dual pack called Diastat acudial with a special delivery system. It has a dial and a lock feature. The pharmacist ensures that the patient gets exactly the prescribed dose. The drug can be administered by rectum after lubricating the nozzle with a lubricating gel. Even if you decide to go to the emergency room, administering this drug at home first would prove very effective in controlling seizures. Your daughter would most likely go to sleep after the administration of the drug. If your daughter has suffered from serious injuries during the seizure(s), has diabetes, has trouble breathing, or continues to have a cluster of seizures without returning back to herself, then you should call an ambulance or transfer her to a nearby hospital. An adolescent with pregnancy and

diazepam (Diastat)
A type of drug used to treat seizures and is administered by anus.

Treatment

seizures should be taken to the hospital as well to make sure that seizure(s) did not have an adverse effect on the fetus.

37. My son had a seizure during school hours. Can you provide me with a medical note with specific recommendations? At what point can he return to school?

There is always a potential chance of having a seizure during school hours. This is more of an issue in children who have not been able to reach optimal control. You should inform the school authorities and the school nurse about your son's medical condition and special needs. Schools typically ask for a doctor's note after any medical illness. The school needs to be made aware of the name of medication(s), tablet strength and frequency, and route of administration. It is not a bad idea to inform some of your son's close friends (if they are old enough to understand) about your son's condition so that prompt help can be rendered. Children and adults have lots of misunderstandings about epilepsy. There is a better chance of teachers or children providing better first aid if they are aware of the seizure type your son has. It may be equally important to discuss how your son behaves right after the seizure. The school does not need to call 911 if the seizure duration is short and he returns to baseline quickly. Someone from the school should call the paramedics if his seizure is unduly prolonged or if he has sustained an injury that requires him to go to the emergency room. I will provide written instructions clarifying the dose of diazepam rectal that needs to be administered by the school nurse in case he gets prolonged seizures. School staff may need special training to use the magnet if your child has a vagal nerve stimulator. (See Part Seven.)

38. What treatment do you recommend for febrile seizures?

Febrile seizures do not require treatment unless they are prolonged or impose risk of status epilepticus (prolonged seizures for more than 30 minutes) or are very frequent. There is no evidence that prophylactic administration of the antiepileptics would prevent development of epilepsy later on in life. Most febrile seizures do not require any long-term treatment with AEDs. However, febrile status epilepticus should be treated as a medical emergency. Intravenous phenobarbital, valproate sodium (Depacon), or diazepam rectal can be used for such emergencies. Parents should be encouraged to use acetaminophen (Tylenol) or motrin to bring the fever down. Tepid sponging can be helpful if the fever shoots up. Bacterial infections should be recognized and treated earlier on to reduce the risk of febrile seizures. Febrile seizures are benign and self-limited.

39. How are infantile spasms treated?

There are several options to treat infantile spasms (ISs). There is no standard care. The first-line treatments include **adrenocorticotropic hormone (ACTH)**, steroids, vigabatrin (Sabril), and pyridoxine (vitamin B_6). The second-line treatments include benzodiazepines, lamotrigine, high doses of topiramate, zonisamide, and divalproex sodium and ketogenic diet.

adrenocorticotropic hormone (ACTH)

A hormone produced by the master pituitary gland; also used in the treatment of infantile spasms.

Adrenocorticotropic hormone has been tried for infantile spasms since it came on the market in 1958. The maximal beneficial effects of ACTH are likely if ACTH is tried early on in the course of the disease. There are two ways to administer ACTH—either as low doses or high doses. We do not have a clear understanding of the optimum dosages or the duration of therapy. Response to ACTH therapy is all or none. It takes about 2 weeks before the benefits are obvious. It not only stops seizures but also improves EEG pattern.

Patients who fail to respond to ACTH may respond to oral high-dose **steroids**. ACTH and steroids can lower the immunity level of your child. Long-term use of either drug is not recommended. Children gain weight, acquire upper respiratory infections, develop acne and increased pigmentation of their skin, high blood pressure, increased glucose levels, and cataracts. The response rates to ACTH or steroids are close to 50–60%.

Vigabatrin (an antiepileptic drug) is the drug of choice in children with tuberous sclerosis. Vigabatrin cannot be used for a long time because of the risk of **toxicity** of the retina—the light-sensitive layer of the eye. Vigabatrin can cause permanent visual field restriction and might not reverse even if the drug is withdrawn. About 30% of patients who take this drug for more than a year develop retinal toxicity. This is one of the reasons that vigabatrin was not approved by the Food and Drug Administration (FDA) in the United States. Visual field changes may or may not be noticed by the patient. Frequent eye examinations are necessary to detect retinal problems. Eye examinations in infants and children may be very challenging. Rarely, vigabatrin can cause facial swelling. Vigabatrin has been tried for partial epilepsy as well, but because of its retinal toxicity, it has never been a first-line drug of choice.

Pyridoxine dependency can cause ISs. Therefore, high doses of pyridoxine are tried in children with IS. The EEG improvement can be seen with intravenous infu-

steroids

Natural or synthetic compounds made of lipid and carbon. Common uses in epilepsy include infantile spasms and Rasmussen's encephalitis in children and girls with worsening of seizures around their menstrual time.

toxicity

Adverse side effects of a drug on a patient.

sion of B$_6$, and the diagnosis of pyridoxine dependency or deficiency can be confirmed. Most of the cases respond in 1–2 weeks. There are several studies showing efficacy of divalproex sodium, newer antiepileptic drugs, or novel therapies such as immunoglobulin or the ketogenic diet in the treatment of IS.

A ketogenic diet can cause 50% reduction in the frequency of spasms. Divalproex sodium, lamotrigine, zonisamide, and topiramate can be tried alone or in combination if initial first-line treatment does not control spasms effectively.

40. What are the side effects of medications?

Most antiepileptic medications share common side effects. **Allergic reactions** that manifest themselves as rashes over the body can be observed. Your child should stop the medication, and you should consult his or her physician. The physician should always look at the rash and advise you further. Not all rashes are drug rashes. Rashes that cause itching are usually milder. Prompt diagnosis, cessation of the offending drug, and early intervention can prevent some other life-threatening rashes such as **Stevens-Johnson syndrome** or **toxic epidermal necrolysis**. These disorders carry a higher mortality rate and involve larger areas of skin and the mucous membranes (e.g., mouth, eyes, genitals). Fortunately, these fulminant rashes occur extremely rarely and may require immediate hospitalization. Other common adverse effects are sleepiness, tiredness, and dizziness. Toxicity may manifest as walking and balance problems, **tremors**, slurred speech, and double vision. **Table 18** lists some of the common side effects of AEDs. Some medicines impair cognition, which may interfere with learning; this is

allergic reactions
Side effects that occur because an individual is sensitive to a drug. One example is a rash.

Stevens-Johnson syndrome
A potentially deadly skin disease usually resulting from a drug reaction. It can involve skin, eyes, and mouth.

toxic epidermal necrolysis
Severe life-threatening skin condition that is characterized by blistering and peeling of the top layer of the skin.

tremor
Involuntary trembling, usually of the hands or head, that can involve the legs, the tongue, or palate.

Treatment

Table 18 Common Adverse Effects of Antiepileptics

Tiredness
Sleepiness
Lack of energy or fatigue
Inability to concentrate
Irritability, behavioral changes, psychosis
Mood changes: anxiety, depression
Changes in appetite: increased or decreased
Weight changes: gain or loss
Nausea, vomiting, diarrhea
Dizziness, blurring of vision, double vision, balance problems, difficulty
   walking
Tremors
Sexual dysfunction

particularly more worrisome in children. However, the continued seizures may have a much more significant negative effect on the brain.

Attention, concentration, and behavioral problems may become an issue with certain medications. Some side effects are dose dependent. That is, as the dose is increased, the side effects are more obvious. It is better to avoid medications that are commonly associated with cognitive side effects, especially in children. Some side effects of drugs are not dose related. These can be unpredictable and are called **idiosyncratic reactions** (see **Table 19**).

Some side effects are genetically predetermined. The drugs are metabolized by the P450 enzyme system in the liver. The liver may not be mature enough during

idiosyncratic reaction

Unpredictable adverse reaction to a drug that is not dependent on the dose or the composition of the drug.

Table 19 Idiosyncratic Side Effects of Antiepileptics

Hypersensitivity reaction (drug rash)
Stevens-Johnson syndrome
Swollen glands
Liver failure and inflammation (not dose dependent)
Bone marrow suppression
Aplastic anemia (anemia where bone marrow stops production of all cell
   lines—white blood cells, red blood cells, and platelets)
Paradoxical increase in the frequency of seizures with antiepileptics

early days of life. The antiepileptics are broken down into compounds that may have toxic effects on various organs **(Table 20)**. The body has its own mechanism to get rid of these toxic metabolites. But some patients have a lack of enzymes that facilitate the removal of toxic metabolites. These patients carry a higher risk of adverse effects to some medications that cannot be detoxified. Asian ancestry is more prone to toxic side effects of tegretol, an antiepileptic drug.

Few antiepileptics are structurally or pharmacologically similar to a certain extent. This may explain why the side effects are common. It also explains how patients can be resistant to several medications. This is termed **medically refractory seizures (MRS)** or **pharmacoresistance**. This term is not precisely defined. This means that the seizures are not under optimal control despite the use of two or three first-line drugs.

There are some long-term side effects of medications. Newer medications are the generation of AEDs approved by the FDA after 1990 (see Question 42). Old or new medications can cause hematological problems. There are three kinds of blood cells in our body: red blood cells,

medically refractory seizures (MRS)

Seizures that are not controlled by medical therapy.

pharmacoresistance

Situation in which medical conditions are refractory to medical treatment.

Table 20   Effects of Antiepileptics on Multiple Organs

Liver: increased liver enzymes, liver failure (rare)
Gastrointestinal: nausea, vomiting, diarrhea
Kidney: stones
Skin: rash, hair growth, hair loss, acne, thickening and coarsening of skin
Eyes: double vision, blurring of vision, glaucoma
Connective tissue: contractures (tightening of skin), lupus-like syndrome
Ovaries: cyst formation (polycystic ovarian syndrome), irregular menstrual cycles
Bones: thinning of bones, decreased mineralization of bones (osteopenia and osteoporosis)
Blood: low white blood cell counts, aplastic anemia (a form of anemia in which the bone marrow stops the formation of red and white blood cells), low platelets, low sodium, low bicarbonate

estrogen

A general term for female steroid sex hormones that are secreted by the ovary and are responsible for typical female sexual characteristics.

progesterone

A steroid hormone produced in the ovary. It prepares and maintains the uterus for pregnancy.

testosterone

A potent androgenic hormone produced chiefly by the testes that is responsible for the development of male secondary sex characteristics.

Any child with a history of prolonged use of antiepileptics should have a bone density test.

Duputyren's contracture

Scar tissue beneath the skin of the palm of the hand. The fingers or sole of the foot can acquire a fixed position. It is commonly seen in patients with epilepsy, diabetes mellitus, and alcoholism.

white blood cells, and platelets. Each has an individual role to play. Medications can preferentially affect any of these three blood lines, or they can affect them all. If all three blood components are affected, this condition is called aplastic anemia; Felbamate can cause aplastic anemia; divalproex sodium can cause low platelets.

There could be electrolyte abnormalities; for example, low sodium or low carbonate may be associated with the use of old or new medications. Antiepileptic drugs may affect the thyroid hormones or sexual hormones such as **estrogen, progesterone,** and **testosterone.** Patients may have gum bleeding or skin and bone abnormalities. Old drugs may be associated with contractures of the skin of palms called **Duputyren's contracture.** Vitamin D and calcium metabolism is deranged with the use of old medications and may have negative impact on the bone health. It is extremely important to supplement calcium and vitamin D to prevent thinning of the bones called osteopenia, which may be associated with risk of fractures or osteoporosis. Any child with a history of prolonged use of antiepileptics should have a bone density test. Risk of osteoporosis is heightened in patients who are immobilized or are physically handicapped, bedridden, or institutionalized. These patients are more likely to be on more than one drug and might not have enough exposure to sunlight. The skin forms vitamin D on exposure to sunlight.

Weight changes are seen with the use of AEDs as listed in **Table 21**. Psychiatric drugs are commonly used in patients with epilepsy and may complicate the picture.

Older medications can be associated with a disease of the nerves; the longest branches of the nerves supplying the feet are affected the most. The longest branches

Table 21 Weight Changes with AEDs		
Possible increase	Possible decrease	Possible neutral
Carbamazepine	Felbamate	Lamotrigine
Divalproex sodium	Topiramate	Tiagabine
Gabapentin	Zonisamide	
Levetiracetam		
Oxcarbazepine		

need the most nutrition. When these nerves are affected, this condition is called **neuropathy**. Folic acid and multivitamin deficiencies can be seen with the use of medications. Over-the-counter multivitamin tablets and folate supplementation are highly recommended in patients on AEDs. See **Table 22** for children's folate requirements.

neuropathy

Disease affecting the nerves that carry different kinds of sensations.

The lower part of the brain, called the **cerebellum**, and which is important for balance and coordination, may shrink, causing balance problems. There are cognitive side effects of antiepileptics. Both old and new antiepileptics share these side effects.

cerebellum

Lower part of the brain that plays a crucial role in maintaining balance and coordination.

41. Are medications harmful to my child's developing brain?

The risks of continued seizures have a worse impact on your child's developing brain compared to some of the cognitive side effects of antiepileptics. Cognitive side

Table 22 Folate Requirements in Infants and Children	
Age	Males and females (micrograms/day)
0–6 months	65
7–12 months	80
1–3 years	150
4–8 years	200
9–18 years	400

effects in children with epilepsy could be multifactorial, and it is not fair to blame medications alone. Impaired cognition could be either due to congenital brain maldevelopment or acquired brain insults such as head trauma, meningitis or encephalitis, or stroke in some children. Hereditary and environmental factors do play a significant role in cognition. Children who undergo successful epilepsy surgery may show improvement in their neuropsychological IQ scores. On the other hand, poorly controlled patients tend to be not only on multiple medications (**polypharmacy**) but, in general, require higher dosages. Higher dosages are frequently associated with higher blood levels. Higher levels have been found to be associated with cognitive impairment. Baseline neuropsychological testing before initiating treatment and repeat testing while on medications can shed more light on the issue of cognitive impairment and drugs. Limited studies done in children have shown very little change in cognitive functioning after medications were discontinued. Barbiturates and benzodiazepines tend to be more sedating and cause more cognitive side effects and should never be the first-line treatment in this most vulnerable period of brain development. Phenobarbital and other drugs of similar class have been associated with irritability, and slowed processing speed.

Since 1990, several newer medications have been approved by FDA to treat epilepsy. The newer medications have few cognitive side effects compared to older antiepileptics. That being said, all clinicians can share their experiences about how the response to treatment and side effects profile differs from case to case. All medications can have behavioral or cognitive side effects. General guidelines may not apply to every indi-

polypharmacy

Use of more than one medication.

vidual case, but use of **monotherapy** (single medication) and low-to-modest dose should be the aim to mitigate cognitive side effects. Early intervention to control seizures in a young child with the lowest number of drugs and lowest dosages is crucial for the child's brain development. Modest cognitive side effects of antiepileptics may be very well balanced out by reduced seizure frequency.

monotherapy

The use of only one drug in the treatment of any medical illness.

42. What is the difference between old and new medications?

More than 10 drugs have been developed by different pharmaceutical companies since the 1990s and have been approved by the FDA. The American Academy of Neurology has defined newer antiepileptics as any antiepileptic approved by the FDA after 1990. Bromides came out in 1857 and were used as antiepileptics until safer drugs were developed. Barbiturates such as phenobarbital and mephobarbital were made available in 1912 and 1935, respectively. The emergence of phenytoin in 1938 revolutionized the treatment of epilepsy, and over the years, phenytoin has emerged as one of the most commonly used antiepileptics in emergency rooms and outpatient clinics. For many decades, not too many antiepileptics emerged until ethosuximide (used for absence seizures) and primidone were approved in the 1950s, and divalproex sodium and carbamazapine came out in the 1960s. Phenytoin, carbamazapine, divalproex sodium, and phenobarbital remained the most commonly used drugs until the 1990s. **Table 23** lists the old and new AEDs. Any drugs approved after the 1990s are called newer **antiepileptics** (see **Table 24**). Response to different medications,

antiepileptics

Medications used to prevent the spread of seizures in patients with epilepsy.

Table 23 Commonly Used Old- and New-Generation Antiepileptics	
Old AEDs	**New AEDs**
Bromides	Felbamate
Carbamazepine	Gabapentin
Divalproex sodium	Lamotrigine
Diazepam	Levetiracetam
Ethosuximide	Oxcarbazepine
Paraldehyde	Pregabalin
Phenobarbital	Topiramate
Phenytoin	Vigabatrin
	Zonisamide

Table 24 New Antiepileptic Drugs			
Year of FDA approval	**Trade name**	**Generic name**	**Pharmaceutical company**
1993	Felbatol	Felbamate	Medpointe
1994	Neurontin	Gabapentin	Pfizer
1995	Lamictal	Lamotrigine	Glaxo-Smith
1996	Topamax	Topiramate	Ortho-McNeil
1998	Gabitril	Tiagabine	Cephalon
1999	Keppra	Levetiracetam	UCB Pharma
2000	Trileptal	Oxcarbazepine	Novartis
2000	Zonegran	Zonisamide	Eisai
2005	Lyrica	Pregabalin	Pfizer

whether new or old, versus tolerance differs from case to case. The physician's main concerns are the following:

- How effective is the drug at controlling seizures?
- What are the side effects?
- How is the overall quality of life on the current medication(s)?

Most medications, whether AEDs or others, are metabolized through the liver. There is an enzyme system in the liver called cytochrome P450 that engages in this metabolism. AEDs can either be P450 enzyme inducers (which enhance the metabolism) or inhibitors (which decrease the metabolism). Newer medications do not have such strong enzyme-inducing or enzyme-inhibiting effects. Levetiracetam and gabapentin completely bypass the liver metabolism. This is certainly more advantageous if the patient being treated has significant liver disease. Absence of liver metabolism means no drug-to-drug interactions. This is particularly helpful in patients who are on **polytherapy**. Physicians aware of these drug-to-drug interactions try to choose a drug with the least drug-to-drug interaction. Newer antiepileptics are less protein bound; therefore, there is more availability of drugs. Some of the older medications shared a common structural compound. This could explain why some patients developed allergic reactions to different AEDs. That being said, drug rash can occur with any drug, new or old. Older drugs with strong P450 enzyme induction enhance the metabolism of vitamin D and increase the risk of osteoporosis of bones with their chronic use. Vitamin D and calcium are important for the deposition of bone minerals and strong bones. Newer medications may prove to be better as far as their effects on bone health are concerned. Patients on older AEDs should be supplemented with calcium and vitamin D. The risk of osteoporosis is lower in children, as active bone formation compensates for the loss of bone, but risk is increased under the following circumstances:

- Female gender
- Sedentary lifestyle
- Thin body habitus
- Caucasian race
- Positive family history of osteoporosis
- Extreme immobilization (e.g., nursing home residents, wheelchair-bound patients)

polytherapy
The use of more than one drug in the treatment of a medical condition.

Treatment

- Drug use (antiepileptics)
- Smoking

Sex steroids such as estrogens, progesterone, and testosterone are metabolized by the liver as well. Newer AEDs might have less interaction with oral contraceptive pills. Any AED that induces the liver enzyme P450 strongly can cause increased metabolism of the sex steroids and thereby lower the efficacy of the birth control pills (see **Table 25**).

Sedation, tiredness, and lethargy are some of the common side effects shared by both older and newer AEDs. However, amongst newer AEDs, lamotrigine and felbamate are considered activating drugs and cause less sedation and fatigue. Overall, lamotrigine is also considered a weight-neutral drug. Felbamate, zonisamide, and topiramate may cause weight loss; this side effect may be welcomed in children who are overweight or teenage girls who are trying to lose some pounds. The decision about choosing an old or new AED or favoring one over the other is also influenced by coexisting **neurological conditions** such as migraine, bipolar or psychiatric disorder, or other medical illnesses.

neurological condition

Medical condition involving the nervous system.

More AEDs were approved to treat status epilepticus using intravenous routes such as fosphenytoin, val-

Table 25 Antiepileptics and Birth Control Pills Interactions	
Mild interactions	No interactions
Carbamazepine	Divalproex sodium
Felbamate	Gabapentin
Oxcarbazepine*	Lamotrigine
Phenobarbital	Levetiracetam
Phenytoin	Tiagabine
Primidone	Zonisamide

*Only at higher dosage

proate sodium, and levetiracetam. Rectal diazepam and buccal midazolam are other choices in treating status epilepticus.

43. I worry about the side effects of medications. What are your thoughts about alternative therapies?

More studies are being done to understand the role of **complementary or alternative therapies**, as 35% of patients with epilepsy do not respond to conventional medical therapy and parents fear the side effects of medications. There are no double-blind randomized drug trials to prove the beneficial effects of complementary or alternative therapies. However, there is a gamut of therapies available out there. NYU Comprehensive epilepsy center has been trying to collaborate with other comprehensive epilepsy centers to evaluate the role of traditional and alternative therapies. About 65–80% of epilepsy patients use traditional medicines worldwide. Asian, herbal, homeopathic, and nutritional therapies are widely used by patients worldwide. **Table 26** lists some of the complementary and alternative therapies used to treat epilepsy.

complementary or alternative therapies

A group of diverse medical and healthcare systems, practices, and products that are not presently considered to be part of conventional medicine.

Asian, herbal, homeopathic, and nutritional therapies are widely used by patients worldwide.

Table 26 Complementary and Alternative Therapies

- Acupuncture
- Aromatherapy
- Ayurveda
- Biofeedback
- Chiropractic
- Herbal medicines
- Homeopathy
- Hypnosis
- Massage
- Meditation
- Nutrition
- Osteopathy
- Yoga

acupuncture

A Chinese tradition in which fine needles are used to stimulate specific areas along certain meridians that balance the energy flow in that area.

St. John's wort

A plant with yellow flowers that is frequently used for depression and anxiety.

ginseng

A medicinal plant of China that is considered a tonic to the whole body.

kava kava

An herbal medicine that comes from a plant native to islands of the South Pacific. It seems to help seizures by increasing inhibition in the brain.

schizandra

Also called *five-taste fruit*, it comes from a woody wine found in Northern and Northeastern China. Schizandra is used to improve mental clarity and to fight depression and stress. It is supposed to enhance concentration and memory.

cod liver oil

Oil that comes from the livers of cod. It is rich in vitamins A and D.

Acupuncture, massage, meditation, hypnosis, music, art, and pet therapies have become the alternative healing resources for several illnesses, including epilepsy. Reflexology, a massage therapy, focuses on the hands, feet, and ears.

Yoga techniques concentrate on relaxation, internal peacefulness, posture, and alignment. This ancient Indian practice that dates back to 2500 BC is now widespread internationally. Yoga combines physical and mental exercise for patients with epilepsy. Exercise has a positive effect in relieving stress and anxiety. Up to one-third of patients find increase in the frequency of seizures during times of stress. Yoga and other forms of exercise are healthy ways to relax. Children with trouble focusing and hyperactivity have demonstrated improved cognitive function after taking up yoga.

Herbal medicines may have herb–drug interactions. Therefore, herbs should be carefully selected as some of the commonly used herbs can worsen seizures. **St. John's wort**, an herbal remedy to treat mild to moderate depression, increases the metabolism and clearance of antiepileptic drugs. A glass of grape juice can inhibit the liver enzyme system and thereby increase the levels of anticonvulsants. **Ginseng**, **kava kava**, and **schizandra** should be avoided in children with epilepsy. **Cod liver oil** should not be taken along with phenytoin. Lots of herbal medicines have heavy metals and other contaminants. Aluminium, arsenic, lead, mercury, tin, and zinc are some of the heavy metals extracted from ayurvedic medicines that can prove harmful to kidneys. A commonly used herb, **gingko biloba (ginkgo)** has been found to decrease the concentration of **gamma-aminobutyric acid (GABA)** that has a protective role in controlling seizures. Ginkgo can worsen seizures by increasing the metabolism of drugs. The levels of phenytoin and divalproex sodium can decrease if these drugs are taken with ginkgo. The quality of these medicines is poorly controlled, and the concentration of different ingredients can vary a lot raising concerns about their safety. Contamination and adulteration have been reported with several unprescribed over-the-counter medications. You must be sure that your child's physician is completely aware of alternative therapies your child is taking.

gingko biloba (ginkgo)

One of the oldest living trees whose leaves are used in the form of a concentrated extract in traditional medicine to improve thinking, learning, and memory.

gamma-aminobutyric acid (GABA)

A neurotransmitter that inhibits neuronal firing.

Treatment

44. What is biofeedback?

Biofeedback is a shortened form of biological feedback and represents the process of recording physiological signals (such as heartbeats) and communicating it in real time to the person from whom it is being recorded. It makes the person aware of internal body states that he or she is not normally aware of through computer, TV, or sounds. The person then uses this information to learn to change the physiology, for example how to lower the heart rate. Other common body functions recorded by biofeedback include blood pressure, muscle tension, skin temperature, and brain waves.

Several specialties in medicine have started to use biofeedback for the treatment of various disorders, and many more are researching its potential. These disorders include epilepsy, high blood pressure, anxiety, incontinence, constipation, migraine and tension headaches, attention deficits, behavioral and emotional problems, difficulty sleeping, pain, irritable bowel syndrome, and more. Therefore, biofeedback can be used not only for seizures but also for the spectrum of other neuropsychological disorders commonly associated with childhood epilepsy. Biofeedback may also be helpful in improving cognitive skills.

For seizures, the physiological monitoring used in biofeedback is done with the help of EEG or monitoring brain waves. The patient is taught how to change the brain waves by learning the mind's effect on the EEG. Many training sessions are usually needed for your child to become more in touch with the mind and body.

One type of biofeedback for epilepsy is called neurofeedback, and it uses training sessions with a computer displaying brain waves to the patient. The display shows the different types of waves, and the patient learns to suppress the waves that are associated more with seizures. The computer provides positive reinforcement when normal waves are produced by the patient and abnormal waves are suppressed. The computer screen prompts individuals to try to alter the direction of the potential—negative versus positive, up versus down. These are referred to as **slow cortical potentials**. The Kotchoubey group studied 52 patients with epilepsy and demonstrated that at least one-third showed improvement in their seizure frequency with biofeedback. The best studied models for clinical neurofeedback focus on sensorimotor rhythm training to reduce seizure frequency and severity. Patients can also be monitored for changes in aura patterns and cognitive function.

Biofeedback for epilepsy has been used for decades, but it is still not common. Another form of biofeedback is by measuring the **galvanic skin response**. In this procedure, electrodes are placed on the patient's palm. With

slow cortical potentials

Negative or positive deflections on the EEG or changes in the magnetic filed in the magnetoencephalogram that last from 300 milliseconds to seconds.

galvanic skin response

Measurement of the electrical resistance of the skin.

alerting, there is an increased facilitation of electricity on the skin. The training is extensive for patient and practitioner, and the sessions are time consuming and may take months to complete. Biofeedback also requires a certain level of patient cooperation and can be expensive. It is not typically covered by health insurance. On the positive side, there are no known side effects and the procedure is not invasive. There are several case series with encouraging results for the use of neurofeedback, but well-designed clinical trials to establish its benefit have not been done. Most of the studies done on biofeedback have recruited a small number of patients and lack supportive evidence in children; further evidence and clinical trials are needed before drawing conclusions about the usefulness of biofeedback in children with epilepsy.

45. I understand the need to control my child's seizures as early as possible. Can my child eventually come off medications?

Parents often raise this question as they are eager to take their child off medications. They have genuine concerns about the short- and long-term side effects of medications. Once an adolescent becomes seizure free for a few months, then they always question the need to stay on treatment. It is natural for a sexually active teenager to worry about the side effects of drugs on female hormones or menstrual cycles, interactions with oral contraceptives, or fears of birth defects in her child in case she gets pregnant. With the emergence of costly antiepileptics, it could simply be a cost issue for some parents, especially those whose children have no health insurance. Some chidren may underreport the frequency of their seizures so that they could still enjoy their freedom, play sports without any restrictions, or still hold on to their driver's licenses.

The decision of taking your child off medications depends on the class of epilepsy your child has. Overall, about 40% of patients would have a relapse within the first year after stopping medications. On the contrary, there are benign childhood epilepsy syndromes, where children outgrow epilepsy and need not be on AEDs for a long time. Febrile seizures do not need to be treated, while febrile status needs aggressive intervention. Any patient with a benign brain tumor or stroke does not need to be on antiepileptics, if he or she has never had a seizure. I recommend treatment after the first seizure if the MRI or EEG is abnormal. There are patients who have partial epilepsies with rare seizures. They may have normal MRIs and EEGs. Once they are put on medications, they may be completely seizure free. The child should be weaned off medications after 2 years of seizure freedom if the MRI of the brain and EEGs have been normal. If the child starts having seizures after the treatment is stopped, I recommend continuation of antiepileptics.

Some of the generalized epilepsies need lifelong treatment. The 2-year rule does not apply for juvenile myoclonic epilepsy patients. They carry a chance of recurrence of almost 100% if taken off medications. About 90% of patients with generalized epilepsy are controlled on low doses of antiepileptics, and the long-term side effects are really not an issue with these patients. Simple lifestyle modifications can go a long way to keep these children seizure free along with medications. Some examples include:

- *Compliance*: take medications on a regular basis
- *Sleep hygiene*: get proper sleep
- *Abstinence from alcohol or recreational drugs*
- *Stress alleviation*: relaxation techniques, controlling anxiety and depression, exercises, music, swimming, and yoga

Young girls and boys should avoid rigorous dieting and diet drugs, as all these lower seizure threshold. They should focus more on eating healthy and staying active.

You and your child must understand the risks and benefits of stopping medications in a particular epilepsy syndrome before doing so.

46. How is status epilepticus (SE) treated?

Status epilepticus is one of the neurological emergencies. Most of the studies done to compare different treatments of status epilepticus have been done in adults. We have extrapolated this adult data information to the pediatric population, which may not be the right approach. A developing brain is very much different from an adult brain. Status can be convulsive or nonconvulsive. In **convulsive** status, convulsions are seen; in **nonconvulsive** status, the patient is seizing in the brain but there is no obvious convulsion seen by the bedside. This is also called **subclinical** status.

Continuous EEG is the only foolproof way to know if a patient is seizing in the brain or not. **Figure 14** depicts EEG tracings of a patient with SE. Nonconvulsive status is hard to recognize without EEG and may just present as coma (prolonged unconsciousness and

convulsive

Caused by or affected with convulsions (violent involuntary contraction or series of contractions of the muscles).

nonconvulsive

Lacking convulsions.

subclinical seizures

Seizures that can only be recognized on the EEG, as patient does not exhibit any abnormal clinical behavior.

Continuous EEG is the only foolproof way to know if a patient is seizing in the brain or not.

107

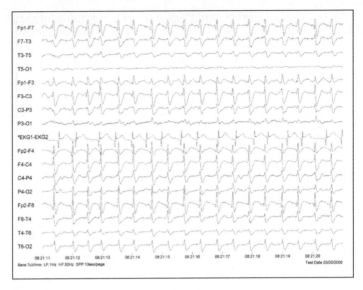

Figure 14
EEG tracings of a patient with status epilepticus. *Source:* Reproduced from Singh A. 2006. *100 Questions and Answers About Epilepsy.* Sudbury, Massachusetts: Jones and Bartlett Publishers, LLC.

inability to respond to any stimuli) or a state of daze or diminished sensibility. It is important to recognize the cause of SE because status is treated as a neurological emergency. **Table 27** highlights some of the complications of SE. Electrolyte imbalances causing status should be recognized and corrected. Infections of the brain such as encephalitis should be recognized by spinal tap, and treatment should be initiated. In several cases, empiric treatment is started with **antibiotics** or **antiviral agents** and stopped once cultures refute the diagnosis of infection. In the epilepsy monitoring units, SE could occur as medications are being tapered to capture seizures. Drug withdrawal SE has a good prognosis and responds to readministration of drugs compared to SE caused by infections of the brain or other brain insults. Pyridoxine deficiency can cause SE resistant to standard antiepileptics. Therefore, it is a standard

antibiotics
Drugs that fight infections.

antiviral agents
Drugs used in the treatment of infections caused by viruses.

Table 27 Complications of Status Epilepticus

Early
- Massive release of stress hormones: risk for heart arrhythmia or cardiac arrest
- Increased heart rate, blood pressure, and blood glucose
- Respiratory failure, fluid in the lungs
- High fever and increased white blood cell counts

Late
- Blood pressure declines—30 minutes or later
- Low glucose, low oxygen, high potassium, low blood volume
- Acute renal failure as a result of lack of blood flow to the kidneys
- Aspiration pneumonia
- Diffuse swelling of the brain

Source: Reproduced from Singh A. 2006. *100 Questions and Answers About Epilepsy.* Sudbury, Massachusetts: Jones and Bartlett Publishers, LLC.

practice to inject 50–100 mg of pyridoxine intravenously for uncontrolled neonatal seizures. EEG abnormalities disappear soon after the intravenous dose. Pyridoxine supplementation is required life-long once the diagnosis is confirmed.

Airway patency, breathing, and circulation need assessment to determine if a patient needs intubation to ensure adequate oxygen supply to the brain. Access to intravenous lines is ensured and saline is infused. Empirical intravenous glucose administration is done to prevent seizures caused by low glucose levels.

Time is a crucial factor in the management of any medical emergency. **Table 28** lists several intravenous drugs used in the treatment of SE. Lorazepam or diazepam rectal should be administered as soon as possible if seizures are unduly prolonged. Intravenous, intramuscular, and per rectal doses are available. Early use of these agents can reduce the morbidity and mortality from status. If patients' seizures do not respond to maximal doses of lorazepam or diazepam rectal, other antiepilep-

Table 28 Treatment of Status Epilepticus
IV lorazepam (ativan)
IV phenytoin (dilantin)
IV fosphenytoin (phosphorylated dilantin)
IV valproate (depakote)
IV phenobarbital
IV levetiracetam (keppra)
Midazolam (versed) IM, nasal, buccal
Continuous IV midazolam infusion*
Continuous IV propofol infusion*
Continuous IV pentobarbital infusion*

*All continuous infusions should be kept on a steady dose for 12–24 hours, and slow withdrawal of infusions is recommended over 24 hours. If seizures return, try even slower withdrawal.

tics are used intravenously. Out of standard AEDs used commonly, only a few can be given by intravenous route for these emergencies. These are phenytoin, fosphenytoin, phenobarbital, divalproex sodium, and levetiracetam. Neonatal SE can be treated with intravenous fosphenytoin or phenobarbital. Fosphenytoin can be given faster than phenytoin. Fosphenytoin is just the modified form of phenytoin (Dilantin). Some small community hospitals do not carry fosphenytoin as it is more expensive. Phenytoin can be given alone or in combination with phenobarbital. These medications are equally effective, but both may be incompletely effective in controlling SE in neonates. Response rate increases to 60% when the two drugs are used in combination. If one of these is given alone, it is able to control seizures in only 50% of neonates. Other therapeutic options are intravenous divalproex sodium or valproate sodium (Depacon). But Depacon is not used in children less than 2 years of age because of their immature liver enzyme system. Valproate sodium may be the first-line treatment for those who have generalized epilepsies or for myoclonic status. Intravenous levetiracetam has been available since July 2006 for use in children older than 4 years of age. We need to wait and watch for its safety in children to treat status epilepticus. However, it is promising that we have more and more alternatives and intravenous antiepileptics.

A child may require intubation to protect the airway if seizures are prolonged and do not respond to diazepam rectal or lorazepam followed by other intravenous infusions. All barbiturates and benzodiazepines can cause low blood pressure and can depress respiratory function. Intubation may be warranted to assist ventilation as higher dosages of medications are being infused to stop seizures. Short or long-acting anesthetics such as propofol, pentobarbital, and midazolam (versed) are used when standard intravenous antiepileptics as mentioned previously fail to stop SE. Parents of children who have a previous history of status epilepticus or who tend to cluster or have prolonged seizures should keep rectal diazepam at home or while traveling. Midazoloam is sold in two other easily used forms, nasal and buccal. Nasal form is a spray absorbed through the lining of the nose. Buccal form is placed against the sides of gums and cheek. These are not approved in the United States but have been shown to be safe and effective in studies done in the United Kingdom and Israel. These forms of midazolam are easier to use, have less social stigma, and are shorter lasting than diazepam rectal.

Surgical intervention, such as hemispherectomy for Rasmussen's encephalitis may be the last resort when all medical therapy fails to control SE. Callosotomy may be offered to children with frequent status and partial seizures with frequent generalization, keeping in mind the complications of status.

Treatment

47. Why are my daughter's medications not working?

About 25–30% of patients have medically refractory seizures (MRS). Any patient who fails more than two anticonvulsants is referred to as refractory, provided the chosen medication was the correct choice for that kind of seizure and the desired dose could be achieved without any tolerance issues. There is a dichotomy observed in children with epilepsy. There are benign syndromes in children that resolve spontaneously and have normal neurologic development. On the other hand, there are catastrophic epilepsies that are associated with mental retardation and are hard to control. There could be several reasons for MRS; a few are mentioned here:

- *Catastrophic epilepsies:* progressive myoclonic epilepsies, symptomatic infantile spasms
- *Types of epilepsy syndromes:* West syndrome, Lennox-Gastaut syndrome, **Ohtahara syndrome**, myoclonic/astatic epilepsy (Doose syndrome)
- *Inborn errors of metabolism:* pyridoxine deficiency, biotin deficiency
- *Brain pathologies:* **cortical dysplasias**, mesial temporal sclerosis, tuberous sclerosis, Sturge-Weber syndrome, arteriovenous anomalies
- *Encephalitis:* inflammation of the brain, especially autoimmune encephalitis such as Rasmussen's encephalitis

Ohtahara syndrome

A catastrophic seizure disorder with onset in newborns. It has different seizure types, such as tonic, partial, or myoclonic.

cortical dysplasia

A malformed, disorganized cerebral cortex.

It is important to revisit the diagnosis of epilepsy and monitor events that are being treated as seizures. The video EEG not only classifies the seizure type but helps to define the epilepsy syndrome and educate more about its prognosis. Certain seizures types such as atonic, tonic, or atypical seizures seen in Lennox-Gastaut syndrome may be very hard to treat. Symptomatic generalized epilepsies or progressive myoclonic epilepsies related to neurodegenerative diseases associated with mental retardation are hard to control even with polytherapy. Abnormal neurological examination or abnormal MRI findings seen in tuberous sclerosis, Sturge-Weber syndrome, or Rasmussen's encephalitis may have a poor prognosis. A few inborn errors of metabolism can have very refractory seizures, such as seizures associated with pyridoxine (B_6) or biotin (B_7) deficiencies.

Resistance to medications has been associated with changed milieu and altered drug transporters. Drugs typically attach to a **transporter** that transports the drug to the target organ in enough concentrations. Two very well recognized drug transporters associated with MRS are **P-glycoprotein** and **multidrug resistant transporter**. In patients with epilepsy, this target organ is the brain. It is believed that there are changes in the brains of patients with MRS. They have overexpression of certain drug transporters, which do not allow enough drug concentrations to reach the target site. These changes could be influenced by long-standing epilepsy as well as the genetic makeup of an individual.

48. I have heard of the use of melatonin in children with epilepsy. I know sleep is important for my son. What is your opinion about melatonin?

Melatonin is a natural product produced by the pineal gland in the brain. No one really knows the exact mechanism of how melatonin works. It is believed to regulate our sleep cycle and works as a biological clock. Sleep is very important for all of us. It helps us rejuvenate from

transporter

Compounds that transport different substances within the body and usually across the cell membranes.

P-glycoprotein

A type of drug transporter protein.

multidrug resistant transporter

These transporters promote the outward flow of drugs away from the site where drugs are needed, and thereby reduce the effectiveness of drugs.

our physical stressors and helps enhance our memory. Melatonin tells our body when to wake up and when to go to sleep. It is maximally secreted at night. Melatonin secretion declines with age. Healthy young adults secrete about 5–25 micrograms of melatonin every night. It can be used to treat insomnia when someone has difficulty falling or staying asleep. There have been small studies in humans where the use of melatonin helped promoting sleep and provided protection against seizures.

Melatonin has not been approved for this indication by the U.S. Department of Food and Drug administration. It is sold as an over-the-counter drug and is available in most health food, grocery, and drug stores. It has been tried in several neurological conditions such as autism, tuberous sclerosis, and Rett syndrome. It is an antioxidant that blocks the bad effects of free radicals. Free radicals are known to cause brain damage.

I would not recommend the use of the natural melatonin because it is made from the pineal gland of animals and could be contaminated by a virus. Synthetic forms are safer. We do not know the long-term effects of melatonin. Melatonin should be given 30 minutes to 1 hour before bedtime. The recommended dose is 3–10 mg. Melatonin is available in 3-mg tablets. I would not recommend this to children who have headaches or depression. Otherwise, melatonin is well tolerated. Most common side effects include headaches, abdominal pain, nausea, and light-headedness. At high doses, the reported side effects include nausea, abdominal discomfort, and diarrhea. It is contraindicated in female patients during pregnancy or breast-feeding.

Your son may be afraid to go to sleep if he has most of his seizures during the night or upon awakening. This is true for patients with frontal lobe seizures, when the child can have a cluster of seizures during sleep. Teenagers tend to have an irregular sleep-wake cycle for several reasons, ranging from lifestyle habits to finishing their school assignments. It should be emphasized that adequate sleep is very crucial. Some very simple sleep tips include:

It should be emphasized that adequate sleep is very crucial.

- Have a regular bed and wake time.
- Engage in a relaxing bedtime activity such as listening to music, reading a book, or taking a nighttime shower.
- Turn off the lights, close the blinds or curtains, and adjust the air conditioning of the room.
- Have a comfortable bed and pillows.
- Use the bed only for sleeping.
- Avoid food 3 hours before retiring to bed.
- Avoid excessive fluids in the evening hours.
- Avoid stimulants such as coffee, tea, soft drinks, alcohol, smoking, etc.
- Avoid vigorous exercise just before retiring to bed.

49. How do you decide that this drug is the right choice for my child?

Once the decision is made to treat seizures with antiepileptics, a single drug is picked. The medications do not cure epilepsy but prevent the spread of seizures and lower seizure threshold. A detailed history of the seizures, as well as an EEG, can help distinguish between partial and generalized seizures. First-line drugs are those that are prescribed alone or used as monotherapy. A second-line drug is added to the first

Treatment

existing drug as an add-on therapy or adjunct if the first drug alone is not effective in controlling seizures. Approximately 70–80% of all patients can be best controlled with a single drug.

Carbamazepine or oxcarbazepine are first-line treatments and for partial epilepsy. Depakote, lamictal, topamax, keppra, and zonegran are frequently used to treat generalized syndromes. The dose should be pushed to the maximum to achieve seizure freedom as long as the patient is able to tolerate the dose. There may be some patients who are unable to tolerate the first medicine because of an allergic reaction or other side effects. If one drug alone fails to achieve seizure freedom for whatever reason, a second-line agent with the least drug-to-drug interaction is tried. The dose of the first agent may need to be adjusted if there are drug-to-drug interactions. The aim is seizure freedom with the lowest possible doses and the least side effects.

50. Are there any new clinical drug trials?

Various trials are under way to find AEDs that control seizures more optimally and with fewer side effects than they currently do. New AEDs are designed and chemically altered to improve safety and tolerability. The National Institute of Health (NIH) and the National Institute of Neurological Disorders and Stroke developed an antiepileptic drug development program in 1974. The antiepileptic drug development program facilitated emergence of laboratories to screen the mechanism of action of drugs. The drug is tested in animal models in these labs; close to 800 compounds are tested each year. Drug trials are expensive; the cost of each new drug that is brought into the market averages about $500 million, taking into account all the failure trials. A new indication may cost an additional $50–100 million depending on whether the antiepileptic drug development program has an elite group of centers perform individual as well as multicenter clinical drug trials. Each drug trial has different phases (discussed next) in the development of a drug until it gets approved or rejected by the FDA.

Phase 0: Trials determine whether a drug behaves in the human body the same way as it did in previous studies. Small doses of drugs are given to a small number of subjects (10–15). This is to determine how the drugs work in the body and how the body processes the drug.

Phase I: About 10–100 healthy volunteers are screened for safety of the drug. In this phase, the drug company focuses on the safe maximum dose and tolerability for 1–1.5 years.

Phase II: About 50–500 volunteers with the disease are studied for close to 2 years. This phase also determines how many patients would go on for a Phase III trial. The possible dose range and preliminary estimates of effective dose is estimated.

Phase III: This phase lasts about 3.5 years. This phase plays a pivotal role in getting FDA approval for the experimental drug. About 3,000 volunteers with the disease enroll in the drug trial to determine the efficacy and adverse side effects of medications, including idiosyncratic reactions.

Phase IV: This phase is also known as a postmarketing surveillance trial. This helps the drug companies to

Treatment

assess the safety of the drug in the long term and in special groups such as pregnant women.

AED trials may require the withdrawal of the previous antiepileptic, or the new AED can be tried as an add-on therapy to the existing therapy. There are direct trials studying monotherapies (new experimental drug versus old drug). Patients awaiting epilepsy surgery can get themselves enrolled in clinical trails. Presurgical and monotherapy trials have patient safeguards and exit criteria that determine when to exit the study.

51. What new antiepileptic is on the horizon?

Lacosamide is a medication developed by UCB to treat partial seizures, which is awaiting approval by the FDA. Retigabine (D-23129) has a unique mechanism of action and works on neuronal potassium channels that help neuronal membrane stability. This drug has completed multicenter trials in 399 randomized patients and proven efficacy in partial seizures with good tolerability in adults. Two pivotal Phase III trials, RESTORE1 and RESTORE2 are currently under way to further investigate the efficacy and safety of retigabine as an adjunctive treatment for partial-onset seizures in patients with refractory epilepsy.

Future approaches include drugs being designed and developed that could work on **M-channels**. M-channels are slowly opening and closing potassium channels that can slow the firing of neurons.

Stiripentol seems to be a promising add-on drug, particularly in combination with carbamazepine in patients with partial childhood epilepsy who are refractory to

M-channels

The slowly opening and closing potassium channels that slow down the firing of neurons and exhibit a net inhibitory effect on the brain.

vigabatrin (VGB) and with clobazam (Frisium) in patients with severe myoclonic epilepsy in infancy.

Gene therapy for epilepsy is still in its infancy but sounds promising as our understanding of **genes** responsible for different epilepsy syndromes is growing. This is an important strategy for introducing genes into the brain, thereby changing the whole milieu in the brain. There is another approach called **cell grafting** that involves brain grafting of cells that are engineered to release inhibitory neurotransmitters or neuroactive compounds.

gene therapy

A technique that corrects defective genes responsible for disease development. A "normal" gene replaces an "abnormal" gene causing the disease.

gene

Hereditary material composed of long strands of four molecules that determine the synthesis of proteins.

cell grafting

A procedure in which stem cells are delivered or transplanted to repair defective machinery in the cells.

52. The medications my daughter is taking are very expensive. Can she take generic drugs instead of brand names?

That is a very intelligent question! It is a hot topic of debate among neurologists and epileptologists taking care of seizure patients. The new generation antiepileptics are being increasingly prescribed by the physicians, and these drugs are much costlier than the old antiepileptics. This becomes an important issue when we consider that more than 9 million children in America are still uninsured. Children of minority groups with a poor socioeconomic background are most at risk. With the rising health costs, there has been an increasing pressure on the hospital pharmacies and insurance companies to promote the less costly **generic drugs** over **brand names**. There are some basic requirements for approval of generic drugs. These should have the same active substance, so they are chemically the same. They are also regulated by the FDA. Generic drugs may come with different colors, sizes, shapes, or names, but their active ingredient, dosage amount, and the route of

generic drugs

Drugs which are produced and distributed after the trademark manufacturers lose their patent protection.

brand name

The name given to a drug by the company that manufactures it.

Treatment

119

administration should be the same. This is called bioe-quivalence. FDA guidelines are strict; a generic drug must have between 80% and 125% bioequivalency to its name-brand product. This is roughly a window of 20% less or 25% greater potency.

The inactive ingredient of the drug may differ. This is also referred to as the vehicle, but this does not affect the most wanted effect of the drug. However, drug levels may vary significantly between the generic and brand names. Most of the generic drugs are not tested in children. There is no particular reason to believe that data available from adult studies can be extrapolated for extremes of age where metabolism of drugs is different.

However, we have had patients who come to us saying they had a breakthrough seizure after they were switched to a generic. One breakthrough seizure may impose restriction to sports-related activities at home or school or expose the child to risk of physical injuries. Some patients complain of more side effects or more seizures with the use of generic drugs. Fortunately, it is not true for the majority of other patients who enjoy spending less money without experiencing seizures or side effects of medications. So there are always concerns but no convincing evidence that generic drugs are associated with increased frequency of seizures and increased side effects.

53. My child cannot swallow tablets. How can I give the medicines?

The majority of young children have difficulty swallowing tablets. AEDs are available in different forms for easy administration to children, such as syrups, chewable tablets, and sprinkles. Valproic acid (250 mg/5 ml), phenytoin (125 mg/5 ml), levetiracetam (100 mg/ml), gabapentin (250 mg/5 ml), carbamazepine (100 mg/5 ml), oxcarbazepine (300 mg/5 ml), and ethosuximide (250 mg/5 ml) are available as syrups. Rectal preparations are available, if your child gets sedated after prolonged seizures or a cluster of seizures. Lamotrigine chewable, dispersible tablets are available by Glaxo-Smith-Kline. Pfizer Inc. makes phenytoin chewable tablets for easy administration. Sprinkle forms are available for divalproex sodium and topiramate. Shire US Inc. makes carbamazepine (Carbatrol) in the form of capsules, with extended-release beads in capsules. An extended-release formulation of carbamazepine is suitable for administration through feeding tubes because the capsules can be pulled apart to release the small granules. One capsule of carbamazepine can be added to the 15 ml of liquid followed by additional 10 ml water flush to avoid blockage of the feeding tube.

54. Should I observe any dietary restrictions for optimal control of my son's seizures?

A lot of parents asks the same question you have asked. Your son does not need any food restrictions. He should eat a balanced diet. In fact, there are certain nutritional disorders responsible for causing seizures. The deficiency of biotin and folate can cause medically resistant seizures.

Your son does not need any food restrictions.

Biotin is involved in several metabolic reactions controlling the metabolism of fats, carbohydrate, and amino acids. Biotin is found in natural foods, and bacteria in the intestines synthesize biotin as well. There could be complete or partial absence of biotin. Severe deficiency signifies less than 10% of the enzyme activity. Children with severe deficiency show disease manifestations in the first 6 months of life. Biotin is broken down to biocytin by an enzyme called biotinidase. The production of biocytin is important for continuous recycling of free biotin. Deficiency of biotinidase causes relative deficiency of biotin. Therefore, both biotin and biotinidase deficiency can cause incalcitrant seizures. Biotin deficiency can cause loss of hair (**alopecia**), developmental delays, hearing and visual loss, acidosis, poor immunity, frequent infections, difficulty walking, and seizures. The seizures can be generalized tonic-clonic, myoclonic, or infantile spasms. This is a very treatable condition, if diagnosed in time. However, delay in diagnosis can cause irreversible neurologic damage, blindness, and hearing loss. Patients on intravenous feeding, **total parenteral hyperalimentation (TPN)** and dialysis patients are prone to development of biotin deficiency. Some children are susceptible to develop biotin deficiency if they eat large quantities of egg whites. Serum enzyme assays can confirm the diagnosis. Children with biotin deficiency do not respond to standard AEDs, but seizures show remarkable improvement with the administration of 10 mg of biotin per day. The pediatric dose varies from 6 to 40 mg/day.

Folate facilitates the synthesis of nucleic acids. Nucleic acids are the building blocks of DNA machinery. Therefore, folate is very important for cell growth and division. Folate is abundant in leafy green vegetables, fruits, dried beans, and peas. Folate requirements for different age groups are highlighted in Table 22. Most of the antiepileptics can cause folate deficiency. Folate defi-

alopecia
Thinning or loss of hair.

total parenteral hyperalimentation (TPN)
The administration of an IV solution to provide complete nutritional support for patients unable to maintain adequate nutritional intake.

ciency can cause anemia, diarrhea, and memory problems. Old antiepileptics frequently cause folate deficiency. It is particularly concerning when women of childbearing age take antiepileptics. Folate deficiency can cause defective formation of the brain and spinal cord in the fetus. These are called **neural tube defects**. Supplementation of folic acid is recommended in all women of childbearing age to prevent neural tube defects.

neural tube defects
Birth defects of the brain and spinal cord.

Vitamin B_6, also called pyridoxine, is an essential cofactor for many enzyme reactions. Pyridoxine deficiency is associated with refractory seizures. Pyridoxine plays an important role in the metabolic reactions leading to gamma-aminobutyric acid (GABA) synthesis. GABA is an important neurotransmitter that inhibits excitation. Pyridoxine dependency is a rare metabolic disorder that can cause neonatal seizures. Children can present with status epilepticus (continuous seizures lasting more than 5 minutes). Other seizure types have been seen with this disorder. Any neonate with hard-to-control seizures is given a dose of pyridoxine 50–100 mg intravenously. Children whose seizures respond well to pyridoxine administration should receive pyridoxine supplements.

55. What is the ketogenic diet?

The ketogenic diet has been accepted as a last resort but effective therapy to treat seizures in children since the 1920s. Most of the data about the ketogenic diet comes from the pioneering work of John Howland and James Gamble from Johns Hopkins University. It mimics the effects of starvation by providing a high-fat, low- to moderate-protein, and very low-carbohydrate diet. The beneficial effects of starvation controlling the seizures can be found in biblical references. After World War II, there was an emergence of the antiepileptic drugs, and the practice of this diet dwindled. There has been a resurgence and interest in the ketogenic diet since the mid-1980s. Despite the emergence of new-generation AEDs, there has not been a significant change in the number of medically refractory cases. Several articles have been published since 1995 looking at the role of the ketogenic diet in children as well as adults.

The brain utilizes glucose primarily as a source of energy. The ketogenic diet is based on the principle that the brain utilizes ketone bodies instead of glucose when glucose reserves are depleted. Ketone bodies are chemicals that are produced under stress or starvation when body fat is burned as an alternative fuel for energy. The diet mimics the effects of starvation or fasting. The ancient Greek physicians treated diseases, including epilepsy, by altering their patients' diet. The diet provides enough energy for activity and growth but avoids excessive weight gain. The body uses fats as its source of energy instead of glucose. But this fat is not completely burned in the absence of glucose (carbohydrates). No one really knows why it works for some children and not for others. The diet has to be properly administered under close supervision of an epileptologist, nutritionist, and pediatrician. The diet has been tried on different seizure types. There can be different ratios of fat to protein to carbohydrates in the ketogenic diet. The classical diet is 4:1—that is, four portions of fat and one portion of carbohydrate and protein. It is believed that the optimal seizure control is likely when fats to carbohydrate/protein ratio is 3–4:1. **Table 29** demonstrates how the ketogenic diet at Johns Hopkins University is intro-

Table 29 Johns Hopkins Protocol to Administer the Ketogenic Diet

- **Before admission**
  Low carbohydrate consumption for 24 hours
  Children examined by the physician
  Fasting starts in the evening

- **Day 1**
  Admitted to the hospital
  Fasting continues
  Fluids restriction (minimally hydrated state is maintained)
  Blood glucose monitored every 6 hours
  Use of carbohydrate-free drugs
  Parents begin educational program

- **Day 2**
  Fasting continues
  Dinner (after 48 hours of fasting); 1/3 of the calculated ketogenic diet
      is given as eggnog given as meal
  Blood glucose checks discontinued after dinner
  Parents begin to check urine ketones periodically
  Small amounts of orange juice are given if extreme ketosis

- **Day 3**
  Breakfast + lunch = 1/3 of the calculated diet as eggnog
  Dinner increased to 2/3 (meal still eggnog)

- **Day 4**
  Breakfast + lunch = 2/3 of diet
  First full ketogenic meal (not eggnog) given at dinner

- **Day 5**
  Full ketogenic diet breakfast
  Sugar-free, fat-soluble vitamin and calcium supplements prescribed
  Prescriptions reviewed, child discharged, close follow-up

duced under careful scrutiny of a dietician and an epileptologist.

A modified ketogenic diet is less restrictive as far as the intake of carbohydrates and proteins is concerned. This improves compliance and has wider choices of meals. Compliance remains the most common reason for dropouts. The diet is difficult to follow. Children may not find food palatable and may have difficulty accepting the strict food restrictions imposed by the diet. The process of measuring and calculating different proportions can be

Treatment

cumbersome for parents. Strict vigilance should be observed constantly so that even small things like sugar in cough syrups or toothpaste are not ignored.

Urine needs to be checked for ketone bodies on a daily basis. A nutritionist keeps a close watch on the child's weight. Children may have a sweetish smell in their breath.

The ketogenic diet has been effective for different seizure types such as myoclonic, atonic, atypical absence, tonic-clonic, tonic, and partial seizures. A Johns Hopkins group has conducted several studies showing the efficacy of the diet over the years. Around 50% of children with epilepsy notice more than 50% reduction in seizures. However, some children drop out because parents find it ineffective or too restrictive.

56. What are the side effects of the ketogenic diet?

Patients on the ketogenic diet may experience side effects. The diet mimics the effects of starvation by providing a high-fat, low-to-moderate-protein, and very low-carbohydrate diet. It provides enough energy for activity and growth. Patients tend to lose weight on this diet. The nutritionist closely observes the weight parameters and makes sure that your child is taking adequate calories. In the initiation phase, the child may suffer from dehydration, nausea, vomiting, and constipation. In the event of dehydration, your child may receive intravenous fluids without dextrose. Fluid restriction is not advised for children taking antiepileptics such as zonisamide and topiramate to avoid dehydration and acidosis. Hypoglycemia (low glucose) is another side effect. The blood sugar is monitored every 6 hours during the initiation phase, and orange juice can be given if sugars are found to be low.

Kidney and gallstones are common in patients on the ketogenic diet. Infections are more common in patients on the ketogenic diet. **Table 30** lists some of the common side effects of the ketogenic diet.

57. Would the Atkins diet help my child's seizures?

The Atkins diet has gained momentum in the last few years. Most of the data about the efficacy of the Atkins diet in epilepsy comes from Johns Hopkins University, Baltimore. Preliminary pilot studies have proven efficacy in medically refractory seizures, but larger studies are required to claim the efficacy of this diet for epilepsy.

Table 30 Complications of the Ketogenic Diet
• Dehydration
• Vomiting
• Constipation
• Low glucose
• Low proteins
• High cholesterol
• High uric acid
• Low magnesium
• Repeated low sodium
• Infections
• Bone thinning
• Kidney stones
• Gallstones
• Acidosis
• Liver or pancreas inflammation (rare)
• Vitamin deficiency
• Mineral deficiency

Treatment

Atkins diet is a low-carbohydrate diet (20 grams/day), but can allow more carbohydrates after initiation. It is combined with high fat intake, just like the ketogenic diet. The only difference is that it is also a high-protein diet; it has no calorie restrictions. Children are discouraged from skipping meals and encouraged to eat three regular-sized meals per day or 4–5 smaller meals. No fruit, bread, pasta, or starchy vegetables are allowed. Dairy products are restricted except cream, cheese, and butter. It is relatively easy to administer and does not require hospitalization during initiation. It is better tolerated, as it is not as restrictive as the standard ketogenic diet. The compliance rates are higher. The preliminary studies show that it has a positive impact in patients when carbohydrate content is less than 20 grams per day. We still need to measure urinary ketones, urinary calcium, creatinine levels, and serum lipids. Early studies on the Atkins diet have been done on a small number of patients. Controlled trials, longer follow-up periods, and long-term safety issues with the Atkins/modified Atkins diet need to be conducted.

PART FIVE

Epilepsy and Other Neurological Conditions

My child who has cerebral palsy has never had any seizures that we are aware of. Should we worry about seizures?

My son has mental retardation. Should we worry about seizures?

My son has involuntary eye blinking without any loss of consciousness. Could these be seizures?

More ...

58. My child has cerebral palsy. His pediatrician sent him to your office for an EEG. He has never had any seizures that we are aware of. Should we worry about seizures?

About one-third of the patients with cerebral palsy have seizures. There are four kinds of cerebral palsy.

1. *Hemiplegic* (hemi = half; plegia = paralysis) *cerebral palsy*—Patients have loss of brain volume in one of the hemispheres. These patients have partial epilepsy. The mean age of onset of epilepsy is around 18 months.

2. *Spastic diplegia*—Most of the children with spastic diplegia are born prematurely. However, it can be found in term infants as well. It is believed that this condition is a result of in utero insult at 28–32 weeks. This is considered the most common type. Epilepsy tends to start around 24 months of age.

3. *Tetraplegic cerebral palsy*—This is the more severe form and the neurologic insult is more diffuse or global. Because the brain insult is diffuse, the patients tend to have generalized seizures. Seizures tend to start at an early age, usually less than 6 months.

4. *Dystonic cerebral palsy*—These patients do not suffer from cortical damage as much as other types do. These children suffer from injury in the basal ganglia (deep nuclei in the brain). Less than 10% of patients suffering from this condition have epilepsy.

If the child is severely affected by cerebral palsy, there is a higher chance of developing epilepsy. Approximately 70% of the patients with cerebral palsy and mental retardation have epilepsy. Epilepsy is more common in tetra- or hemiplegic types than dystonic or diplegic cerebral palsy.

These patients have multiple seizure types, and prolonged status epilepticus is more likely to occur. The seizures can be refractory to treatment. These patients are on multiple drugs and are more prone to lifelong side effects of antiepileptics. Seizures in these patients are poorly described and not properly witnessed. Most of these patients are institutionalized. Sometimes, it is hard to tease out the difference between the real seizures and the other stereotypes such as self-stimulating behavior, muscle spasms, and tics. Video EEG becomes the gold-standard diagnostic test to clarify the doubts about atypical episodes.

Seizures in these patients are poorly described and not properly witnessed.

59. My son has been recently diagnosed with mental retardation based on IQ testing. What could be the reasons? He was normal at birth. Should we worry about seizures?

Epilepsy is commonly associated with mental retardation. Mental retardation (MR) is based on intelligence quotient (IQ). To measure IQ, we first need to know the mental and chronological age of the person. Chronological age is measured by the time (years and months). Mental age is the actual intellectual development as measured by an intelligence test. A 6-year-old could be performing at a mental level of 8 years old. Another child might be 10 years old but performing at a mental level of 7 years old. IQ is the ratio of 100 times the mental age (MA) to chronological age (CA).

$$IQ = 100 \, MA/CA$$

Approximately 3% of the population has MR, and about 10–20% of all mentally retarded or developmentally delayed children suffer from epilepsy.

Mental retardation is classified into four types, based on your child's intelligence quotient (see **Table 31**).

IQs have a wide range, typically from 0 to 200, although children can have an IQ above 250. About 80% of the general population has an IQ of 80–120. Severe MR is recognized early on during infancy and childhood. Children with mild MR may go unnoticed until they enter school. IQ test is instrumental in educational counseling, and help us understand the psychological and psychiatric issues. There are several causes of mental retardation.

- Genetic
- Phenylketonuria
- Fragile X
- Down syndrome
- Rett syndrome (in girls)
- Low birth weight
- Lack of oxygen at birth
- Cerebral palsy
- Trauma
- In utero insults
- Infections acquired after birth
- Tuberous sclerosis (60% of tuberous sclerosis patients have MR)
- Neurofibromatosis
- Sturge-Weber syndrome
- Folate deficiency
- Iodine deficiency

Table 31   Types of Mental Retardation with respective Intelligence Quotient

Types	Intelligence Quotient
Mild	50–70
Moderate	35–49
Severe	20–34
Profound	Less than 20

The prevalence of MR is about 0.3–0.8%. MR is seen in about one-third of children with epilepsy. About 8% of children with MR develop seizures by the time they turn 5 years old. MR patients are unusually susceptible to the adverse behavioral side effects of all medications. Patients with severe or profound MR are unable to express the side effects. Subtle changes listed here could serve as clues to drug toxicity.

- Altered sleep pattern
- Self-stimulation
- Aspiration
- Drooling
- Irritability, increased restlessness
- Changes in neurological status (deterioration)

Table 32 shows the prevalence of children with mental retardation and/or cerebral palsy who also have epilepsy.

Table 32   Epilepsy in Special Populations of Children

Disease	Association with epilepsy (percentage)
Children with mental retardation (MR)	10%
Children with cerebral palsy (CP)	10%
Children with MR and CP	50%

60. My son has involuntary eye blinking without any loss of consciousness. His pediatrician wanted me to get an EEG. I doubt these are seizures. What do you think?

You are correct. I think the movements he is having right now are not seizures. I think these are simple **tics**. Tics are involuntary movements that are more common in boys than girls. These tend to occur before adulthood. Tics can be simple or complex. Tics can be motor or vocal. Rapid eye blinking, tensing the abdomen, touching the ground, sniffing, throat clearing, grunting sounds, complex movements, and inappropriate words are some examples of tics. Motor tics can affect any part of the body. Anxiety and stress can make these involuntary movements worse. Sleep decreases the frequency of tics or any other movement disorder. Patients have the urge to make these movements, but they can partially suppress the movements, unlike seizures. Suppression of movements can cause uneasiness and discomfort. These can make the person slow, as tics can be disruptive. Tourette's syndrome is a type of tic disorder with vocal-motor tics. Most children with Tourette's syndrome start having tics between 3 and 10 years of age. The worst tics are seen between 9 and 13 years of age. About 50% of the children with tic disorder can have **obsessive-compulsive behavior**. They are heard saying obscene words or socially inappropriate remarks. This is called **coprolalia**. Children suffering from tics might repeat words said by others, called **echolalia**. They may even imitate another's movements, called **echopraxia**. Children with Tourette's syndrome have attention-deficit hyperactivity syndrome and learning difficulties. Tics are not under your child's control. It is understandable that these movements can be embarrassing, espe-

tics

Repetitive motor or vocal movements or a combination of both that is difficult to control.

obsessive-compulsive behavior

An anxiety disorder characterized by recurrent, persistent obsessions or compulsions. Compulsions are repetitive, purposeless behaviors that the individual generally recognizes as senseless and from which the individual does not derive pleasure.

coprolalia

Involuntary utterance of obscene and inappropriate words.

echolalia

Repetition of spoken words by another person.

echopraxia

Imitation of the observed movements of another.

cially in public places. Children try to avoid school to avoid embarrassment in front of classmates. Parents should never ask the child to suppress the movements. Most tics are self-limiting and should not be treated unless these cause discomfort. Several medications, including atypical antipsychotics, baclofen, benzodi-azepines, clonidine, fluphenazine (Prolixin), guanfacine (Tenex), pergolide (Permax), and pimozide (Orap) may be useful in treating tics. **Habit reversal therapy (HRT)** is a kind of behavior therapy that causes significant reduction in tics. HRT includes awareness and relaxation techniques. The child is taught to antagonize the movement caused by a motor tic. This is called competing response. It is done for about 3 minutes after each tic.

habit reversal therapy (HRT)

A behavior therapy used in the treatment of tics.

61. My son is very hyperactive compared to other children of his age. His school teachers have been complaining about his inattentiveness at school. What can be done about it?

It sounds like your child may have a condition called **attention deficit/hyperactivity disorder (ADHD).** ADHD has two core components, inattention and hyperactivity/impulsivity; diagnosis is made if both components last more than 6 months. Either component can occur independently or they can present in a combined form. ADHD is seen in 3–7% of school-age children in the United States. About 60% of children with Tourette's syndrome also suffer from ADHD. ADHD has 3–11% prevalence and is at least twice more common in boys than girls. It is much less prevalent in Europe and Japan. About 30–50% of children with ADHD seem to suffer from other neuropsychiatric con-

attention deficit/ hyperactivity disorder (ADHD)

Neurobehavioral disorder characterized by the symptoms of hyperactivity, impulsivity, and attentional deficits.

ditions and neurobehavioral disorders. Depression and anxiety disorder can coexist. Children develop social phobias and can exhibit obsessive-compulsive or oppositional-defiant behavior.

Genetic causes seem to play the major factor in causing ADHD. Relative lack of dopamine (a neurotransmitter in the brain) in the frontal lobe has been incriminated as a cause of ADHD.

Children suffering from attention deficit/inattention disorder have difficulty sustaining concentration. Children have difficulty focusing on the relevant stimuli and get easily distracted by irrelevant stimuli. They make careless mistakes and have poor organizational skills. They face problems focusing on one particular task. These children take an unusually long time to finish a task or leave it unfinished. They are forgetful and do not finish or submit their school assignments on time. This inattention may or may not be complicated by hyperactivity.

hyperactivity/impulsivity

A state or condition of being excessively active.

Hyperactivity/impulsivity makes a child very fidgety, anxious, and restless. Children with this disorder have difficulty staying still. They may even walk out of the classroom or fail to follow the norms or discipline in the classroom. This kind of behavior can be very disruptive during classroom sessions and can lead to academic underachievement or require placement in special education schools.

Neuropsychological testing can help assess the brain's ability to process feedback, interpret events, and judge mental skills. Children with ADHD tend to have problems with continuous performance tests, working memory, and understanding. Impulsivity can be checked by special timed computer tests. Connor's rating scale is used commonly to diagnose ADHD in children over 6 years of age and adolescents. The revised teacher, parents, and self-reporting scales are available in short and long formats, which help make a diagnosis and monitor the effectiveness of drugs in controlling various symptoms.

Absence seizures, vision and hearing problems, sleep apnea, developmental and learning problems, or language delays should be considered and excluded in a child with possible ADHD. Use of medications or recreational drugs and some mood and anxiety disorders can resemble ADHD.

In the last decade, there has been a surge of new medical therapies for the treatment of ADHD. Commonly used drugs are listed in **Table 33**. Two main stimulants—

Table 33 Drugs Used for ADHD	
Types of Stimulants	**Examples of drugs**
Short-acting stimulants	Methylphenidate, dexmethylphenidate (Focalin), amphetamine/detroamphetamine (Adderall), dextroamphetamine (Dexedrine), amphetamine (Dextrostat)
Intermediate-acting stimulants	Methylphenidate SR, dexmethylphenidate ER, methylphenidate hydrochloride (Metadate) ER, methylphenidate LA, methylphenidate hydrochloride CD, dextroamphetamine
Long-acting stimulants	Methylphenidate, amphetamine/dextroamphetamine XR, dexmethylphenidate XR
Adjuvants to stimulants	Clonidine (Catapres), Guanfacine
Alternatives to stimulants	Atomoxitine (Strattera), bupropion (Wellbutrin), tricyclic antidepressants
Long-acting prodrug stimulants	Lisdexamphetamine dimesylate (Vyvanse)

The side effects of stimulants have not been studied in patients younger than 6 years of age.

methylphenidate (Ritalin) and dextroamphetamine (Dexedrine) are the mainstay of treatment. Short-acting formulations are effective only for 3–5 hours. The effects of intermediate-acting stimulants can sustain the beneficial effects for 6–8 hours. Long-acting formulations are now available, allowing a single-dose schedule; their beneficial effects last up to 12 hours. If a long-acting drug is unable to sustain the beneficial effects, a short-acting stimulant can be added in the early evening hours. Patients notice trouble sleeping and problematic effects on evening appetite with long-acting formulations. The side effects of stimulants have not been studied in patients younger than 6 years of age. The child's appetite, weight, and blood pressure parameters have to be observed carefully. These medications should not be taken on an empty stomach. Stimulants can sometimes exacerbate tic disorders. It is advised to use stimulants with caution in children suffering from tics.

Pellets/beaded capsules can be opened and sprinkled on food. Parents find omega-3 fatty acids and fish oil to be effective in controlling the hyperactivity and impulsivity.

Rett syndrome

An inherited disorder exclusively found in girls that is characterized by brief normal development followed by cognitive decline, loss of developmental skills, autistic features, balance problems, and loss of purposeful hand use.

MECP2 gene

A gene that is important for the function of nerve cells and important to form connections between the neurons (synapses). Defective copy of this gene is responsible for Rett syndrome.

62. My daughter has seizures, autism, and developmental delays, and sometimes she makes abnormal repetitive, purposeless hand movements. I am not sure if the hand movements are seizures as well. How can I tell?

Your daughter may have a condition called **Rett syndrome**. It is a genetic syndrome that exclusively affects young girls. The mean age of onset is around 48 months. Changes in the **MECP2 gene** at X-chromosome 28 cause the disease. CDKL5 gene mutation has been associated with Rett syndrome. With MECP2 mutation, the risk of seizures is higher during the first 4 years of life; this risk decreases after 4 years of age. Children acquire early milestones normally. Girls typically develop normally in early infancy. Gradually motor and language developmental delays, regression of developmental milestones, and autistic behavior draw the attention of parents. Girls often have stereotyped purposeless movements and other repetitive behavior such as teeth grinding or babbling. There are different clinical and EEG changes in different stages of the disease. The four stages of Rett syndrome are described here:

1. Early onset stagnation stage
2. Rapid destructive stage
3. Pseudostationary stage (false impression of being stationary or stable)
4. Late motor deterioration stage

Seizures occur in up to 80% of patients. Major seizure types include tonic, atonic, absences, atypical absences, and complex partial seizures. Myoclonic and infantile spasms can occur as well. It is important to make a distinction between seizures and other stereotypical behaviors such as blank stare and apnea (difficulty breathing). See **Table 34**.

Table 34 Stages of Rett Syndrome		
Stages of Rett syndrome	Clinical Symptoms	EEG
Stage I	Normal development	Normal or minimally slow
Stage II	Autistic features Stereotypical behaviors	Loss of normal awake and sleep rhythms Epileptic activity
Stage III	Seizures Balance problems	Increase in epileptic discharges (generalized; multifocal)
Stage IV	Severe disability Scoliosis	Persistence of epileptic activity

63. My child was recently diagnosed with autism/pervasive developmental disorder. What could have caused this condition, and can he develop epilepsy?

autism

A developmental disorder that impairs communication and social skills.

Autism is an impairment of social and communication skills that sets in before the age of 2 or 3 years. Poor eye contact, lack of social smile and social play, speech delays, and unusual behaviors should raise suspicion for the disease. Researchers have found that autism may involve a lack of coordination in separate areas of the brain. High-functioning autistic kids can outrival others at details but may miss the larger picture. It could be that the cabling system of the brain is at fault. Autism affects 2 to 6 per 1,000 children. Children with the following risk factors may be at an increased risk:

- Prematurity
- Low birth weight
- Breech presentation (head-up instead of normal head-down presentation at birth)
- Low Apgar scores (a score given to a newborn at 1 and 5 minutes after birth)
- Family history of autism or autistic spectrum disorder
- Family history of language delays
- Family history of psychiatric disorder (psychoses, bipolarity, and depression)

Other factors that have been linked with a slight increased risk of autism include mother's health and prenatal care during pregnancy, German measles infection in early pregnancy, difficult labor, and older age of the father. Sudden increase in the head size in the first year of life may be an early indicator after birth. Autism affects various parts of the brain and can be mild or severe. Some examples include autistic disorder, **pervasive developmental disorder** and **Asperger's syndrome (AS)**.

Children with Asperger's syndrome might have some features of autism but have normal intelligence and intact language. However, these children have poor social skills. There is an increased risk of epilepsy in patients with autism. Common neurological disorders associated with autism and epilepsy include tuberous sclerosis, infantile spasms, and Landau-Kleffner syndrome.

64. My son's pediatrician suspected an inherited metabolic disorder but could never come up with a definitive diagnosis. Can you do more tests that haven't already been done to find out what is wrong with my child and his prognosis?

Inherited metabolic disorders (IMDs) are disorders in the metabolism of carbohydrates, proteins, and fats. Carbohydrates, proteins, and fats serve as energy fuels for our bodies. The food that we eat gets broken down into various substances. Various enzymes and coenzymes carry out chemical reactions. These are commonly known as **urea cycle**, **amino acid**, and **organic acid disorders**. The defects in these steps of metabolism—complete absence or partial deficiency of enzymes or coenzymes—can cause accumulation of toxic substances in the body that are harmful to the brain or other organs. Lysosomal and glycogen disorders are examples of so-called **storage diseases** that can pres-

pervasive developmental disorder

Broad term includes autism, Rett syndrome, Asperger's syndrome, childhood disintegrative disorder, and atypical autism.

Asperger's syndrome (AS)

Disorder characterized by stereotyped behaviors and difficulties in social interaction without delay in language.

inherited metabolic disorders (IMDs)

IMDs include defects in the metabolism of proteins, carbohydrates, and fats from birth.

urea cycle disorders

Urea cycle is a cycle of biochemical reactions that produces urea from ammonia. Deficiency of enzymes in the urea cycle can cause increased levels of ammonia.

amino acid

An organic molecule that forms proteins in living organisms.

organic acid disorders

Congenital metabolic disorders where specific enzymes are absent resulting in accumulation of organic acids in blood and urine.

storage diseases

Neurological disorders affecting various parts of central and peripheral nervous system and other organs where too much of a substance, such as fats or enzymes, builds up in the brain and other organs.

ent with enlarged heart, spleen, and liver. Commonly inherited metabolic and genetic diseases include:

- Disorders of carbohydrate metabolism
- Amino acid disorders
- Organic acid disorders
- Lysosomal disorders
- Peroxisomal disorders
- Mitochondrial disorders

Clinical diagnosis is difficult because of the overlapping symptoms in several disorders. IMDs are suspected when there is developmental delay; feeding and breathing problems at birth; or recurrent episodes of vomiting, seizures, and lethargy. Onset of symptoms may coincide with starting feeds or changes in diet. Seizures may occur before the infant is born. Seizures in the uterus could be misperceived by the expecting mother as increased fetal movements.

Careful physical and neurological examination is very helpful in suspecting an inherited condition. Involvement of the skin, nails, muscle and nerves, vision, and hearing problems make your child's physician think of a plethora of inherited diseases. Some defects become obvious at birth when an infant has to digest breast milk or bottle feeds. Abnormalities in the brain may be obvious at birth or appear later on as the brain develops. These disorders present with developmental delays, learning difficulties, seizures, or vision and hearing problems. Weakness, walking problems, and skin involvement could be the hallmark of several IMDs. More than one family member could be affected. Marriages between close relatives, called **consanguineous**

consanguineous

Descended from the same ancestor as another person.

marriages, are responsible for transmission of defective carrier genes from both parents resulting in a few IMDs. Certain races and ethnic groups are susceptible to a group of inherited metabolic diseases. **Ashkenazi Jews** carry defective genes for several inherited metabolic and genetic disorders. **Mitochondrial disorders** are another class of genetically inherited diseases related to mitochondria. **Mitochondria** are power houses of a cell that power most cell functions. Muscles, brain, and nerves requiring most of the energy get affected the most in these disorders. Genetic counseling should be provided to families in these high-risk groups.

Hearing and vision examination should be conducted in all children. Blood, urine, blood gas, ammonia levels, spinal fluid, tissue biopsy (skin, liver, muscle, nerve biopsies) are frequently ordered tests to understand the nature of IMDs. Measurement of enzyme levels and MRIs and EEGs are important diagnostic tests. Lactate and pyruvate levels in the blood and spinal fluid are measured to detect mitochondrial disorders. Newborn screening is available for some IMDs. **Tandem mass spectroscopy,** a technique used since the 1990s to screen newborns for inherited disorders, can detect some of the IMDs. Children may develop normally and the neurological symptoms may appear late. Early diagnosis before the onset of symptoms can improve overall prognosis. Failure to recognize the disease and provide appropriate intervention can cause permanent neurological sequelae. Chromosomal analysis and genetic testing can help confirm the diagnosis.

Treatment revolves around correcting the metabolic defect. Vitamin supplementation can help seizures in

Ashkenazi Jews

Jews descended from the medieval Jewish communities of the Rhineland.

mitochondrial disorders

Group of disorders related to diseases of the mitochondria.

mitochondria

Cellular energy sources.

tandem mass spectroscopy

A tool used for measurement of molecular mass of a sample. This technique is used to understand the composition of proteins, drug metabolism, neonatal screening, and drug testing.

Epilepsy and Other Neurological Conditions

enzyme replacement therapy

A medical treatment that focuses on supplementing an enzyme in patients where the enzyme is partially or completely absent.

bone marrow transplantation (BMT)

Transplantation of the blood cell lines found in the bone marrow from person to person or patients' own bone marrow cells after pretreatment.

Landau-Kleffner syndrome (LKS)

A rare childhood syndrome in which the child has seizures and regression of language.

acquired epileptic aphasia

Regression of language after normal language development.

verbal auditory agnosia

Inability to understand spoken language without any hearing problems.

aphasia

Language disorder resulting from damage to portions of the brain that are responsible for language.

agnosia

Loss of ability to recognize objects, people, shapes, smells, or sounds.

conditions such as biotin and pyridoxine deficiency states. Folinic acid responsive seizures can be associated with intractable seizures resistant to most AEDs, but can be treated with folinic acid. Vitamin supplementation can reduce the frequency of seizures and other neurological complications. One such example is coenzyme Q10 deficiency. Restriction of certain diets can be helpful in the treatment of amino acid, organic acid, and urea cycle disorders. **Enzyme replacement therapy** is used for some metabolic disorders, making up for the deficient enzyme. **Bone marrow transplantation** can be helpful to treat some of the white matter diseases called leukodystrophies. Gene therapy that corrects defective genes responsible for a disease state is also available for IMDs.

65. My child was diagnosed with significant speech delays. I was referred to you by a speech therapist to rule out epilepsy. I am not sure why. Can you tell me?

This could be **Landau-Kleffner syndrome (LKS)**. LKS is also known by other names such as **acquired epileptic aphasia** and **verbal auditory agnosia**. **Aphasia** or **agnosia** in this context means loss of ability to understand written or spoken language. A child starts to learn a language, but then there is a rapid reduction in spontaneous speech. This is called regression of language. Motor development is normal. Language makes us different from nonhuman primates. In humans, language is primarily a function of the left side of the brain. An EEG on children with aphasia or agnosia can be abnormal, especially during sleep.

There may be **continuous spikes and waves during slow sleep** or **electrical status epilepticus of sleep**. In simplified words, the EEG can be very abnormal and show lots of epilepsy brain waves. ACTH, clobazam, and lorazepam have been tried to suppress the electrical status. Sleep, especially deep sleep, activates the EEG. Children with LKS can have different seizure types such as atypical absence, tonic-clonic seizures, or partial seizures. Atypical absence may precede the complex partial seizure. The peak age of onset of seizures is between 4 and 5 years. Seizures tend to occur in the night. Seizures can remit by adolescence. The neuropsychological functioning can show global delays in a child; more specifically, the child might have speech delays. The EEGs can show frontal or temporal focus. Anticovulsants, steroids, speech therapy, and **neurosurgery** are different treatment modalities to improve language function. One-third of LKS patients continue to have severe impairment in language despite all interventions.

LKS has to be distinguished from its variants such as **autistic epileptiform regression** and **disintegrative epileptiform disorder**. Autistic epileptiform regression is recognized by an earlier age of onset (between 1 and 3 years). Salient features of autism, such as lack of social and communication skills along with behavioral problems (e.g., rage outbursts and increased motor restlessness) and cognitive impairment are seen in autistic epileptiform regression. Disintegrative epileptiform disorder displays a severe degree of mental retardation along with mood swings, hyperactivity, and difficulty sustaining attention and concentration. Continuous spikes and waves during slow sleep are considered

continuous spikes and waves during slow sleep (CSWS)

Abnormal EEG findings in an acquired language disorder called Landau-Kleffner syndrome.

electrical status epilepticus of sleep

An EEG pattern showing significant activation of epileptiform discharges in sleep.

neurosurgery

Surgery that is carried out for the treatment of conditions of the nervous system.

autistic epileptiform regression

Global delays in language and social skills in the second year of life after normal development in the first year.

disintegrative epileptiform disorder

This disorder tends to occur between the ages of 2-10 years in autistic children. Children with this disorder can have clinical seizures or abnormal EEG. Children tend to have behavioral issues such as trouble with attention and, concentration, mood swings or cognitive issues.

another LKS variant. Children with LKS but without continuous spikes and waves during slow sleep have more focal EEG abnormalities especially in the left (language) areas.

PART SIX

Miscellaneous

When can my son return to school after a seizure?

My son has a driver's learner permit. He has not had a seizure for the last 2 months. Can he drive?

My son is very athletic. What sports activities can he participate in? Can he swim or scuba dive?

More ...

66. When can my son return to school after a seizure? Should I inform the school?

If your child feels back to normal, there is no need to skip school the next day. However, it is important that you as parents communicate with the school staff. You should try to educate yourself about seizures. You, your son, and his or her close peers can meet and have a more open discussion about the warnings, symptoms, and risk of injuries so that the staff is prepared to handle any such emergencies in the school with a better understanding of his needs. Adapting to new lifestyles or simply returning to sports with due precautions may need to be discussed with your physician, your son, and his coaches. Schools may ask for a doctor's note stating your son's condition, drugs administered, and their dosages (if he is taking any AEDs during school hours) or any lifestyle limitations. Cyberonics Company, manufacturers of vagal nerve stimulators, has support and educational programs in school, residential, and group homes. Cyberonics educational outreach programs can help training school staff and nurses to swipe a magnet in the event of a seizure at school. The nurses should be notified if your child has been recommended to have diazepam per rectum for a cluster of seizures or prolonged seizures. A few children with very frequent seizures may not be able to attend school until their seizures are under better control. Schools have provisions to provide such children with home tutoring, if they receive a supporting letter from their physician.

67. My son has a driver's learner permit. He has not had a seizure for the last 2 months. Can he drive?

Those who are 18 years old or older can drive if their seizures are well controlled. You should contact the department of motor vehicles (the name of the department may vary in your state) to know the rules and regulations in your state. The requirements for different states vary but on an average require 6 months to 1 year of seizure freedom before someone with epilepsy is allowed to drive. The DMV can allow your son to drive under exceptional circumstances such if he has simple partial seizures only without impairment of consciousness, or if he has exclusively nighttime seizures. You have to understand that driving is a privilege, not a right. About 8.5–13.5% of drivers with epilepsy have one or more motor vehicle accidents. Tough rules and regulations are mandatory for the safety of your son, other vehicle operators, passengers, and pedestrians. About half of seizures that happen while driving result in crashes. The crashes can also be the result of medication-related reflex slowing, cognitive impairment, or incoordination. Patients with uncontrolled seizures pose a serious threat on the road, just like those who are driving while intoxicated. Your son's physician may be required to submit a supporting letter explaining his seizure freedom, **compliance**, adequate follow-up, and the reliability of his antiepileptic levels. It is prudent that he report his seizure frequency honestly to his physician. However, it is your state's regulations committee that is responsible for implementing the laws that grant him permission to drive. California, Delaware, Nevada, New Jersey, Ore-

compliance
Taking medications as prescribed.

gon, and Pennsylvania are the only six states that require physicians to report if patients are still having seizures. State laws have not been defined very clearly in regards to epilepsy and driving. A physician's opinion is given consideration, but the department of motor vehicles' medical advisory board makes a final decision. Sleep deprivation, alcohol provocation, and stress are common causes of breakthrough seizures in most epilepsies. One very simple piece of advice is to not drive if you do not feel well rested.

68. My son is very athletic. What sports activities can he participate in? Can he swim or scuba dive?

He can ride his bicycle or use in-line skates, but he should wear a helmet. I would encourage your son to swim. However, there should always be some kind of supervision. Encourage your son to swim during pool hours when a lifeguard is available. The lifeguard should be made aware of your son's condition. An adult who is a good swimmer can supervise him in the pool. Encourage your son to swim in shallow water where an adult could do one-to-one supervision and where your son can stand easily with his mouth and nose out of the water. Your son should swim with other swimmers who should be made aware about his medical condition. These swimmers should be strong enough to save your child, in the event that a seizure happens while swimming. It might be worthwhile avoiding swimming in deep or murky water.

Children with tonic seizures are at a higher risk of drowning early. During a tonic seizure, the muscles of the chest wall contract and air gets expelled from the lungs. This results in higher body density than the density of the water, causing submersion. The relaxation of the chest muscles allows water to go into the lungs, further complicating matters, and the child might not get a chance to emerge from the water. I would not recommend swimming in the sea, as high tides can jeopardize your son's safety in the event of the seizure, and the supervisor might not have enough time to save him.

You should not stop your son from participating in sports just because of epilepsy. That being said, limitations on certain sports activities (see **Table 35**) should be observed. The degree of required supervision varies on individual factors. The seizure type and the frequency of seizures have an important bearing on the precautions observed or the restrictions imposed on your son's sports activities. If your son has seizures clustered during nighttime or a few hours after waking up, you should not be dwelling on his safety while playing sports. He might not be vulnerable during daytime. There are other children who clearly experience warning symptoms that allow them to stop the sports activities. All popular sports activities—such as baseball, basketball, football, tennis, soccer, hockey, golf, wrestling, and running—at different leagues or schools are very closely supervised.

Table 35 Sports to Be Avoided by Patients with Seizures

Underwater swimming
Scuba diving
High diving
Hang gliding
Mountain climbing
Flying
Parachuting
Car racing

Coaches must be properly informed about your son's seizure disorder. *Take due precautions but do not overprotect him.* Use of helmet can prevent serious head injuries. You do not want your child to lose confidence or ability to perform day-to-day activities. Encourage your child to live as normal a life as possible.

Scuba diving should not be allowed until he is seizure free and off medications for more than 5 years. Scuba diving is a particularly risky sport. There are many stimuli (rapid breathing, flickering lights, increased partial pressures of oxygen or oxygen toxicity, exposure to gases at depth, breathing oxygen under increased pressures, low temperatures) involved with diving that are known to lower the seizure threshold. The **Divers Alert Network**, a nonprofit organization since the 1980s, and the Professional Association of Diving Instructors have been promoting educational programs and research that promote safe diving. I would not advise him to scuba dive while on medications. Seizure medications that frequently cause drowsiness enhance the chances of nitrogen narcosis even at shallower depths. Seizures are unpredictable, and it is hard to quantify with confidence the risk of recurrence after a prolonged period of remission. As a parent, you have to understand the risks involved with scuba diving. If your son has not had a seizure for more than 5 years, then he can be permitted to dive under shallow depths, not more than 10 meters. A full face mask is preferred over a regulator, which is a device kept in the mouth by clenching the teeth. Nitrox (an oxygen-enriched mixture with less nitrogen than air) should be avoided.

This 5-year rule is relaxed under the following circumstances:

Divers Alert Network (DAN)

It is a nonprofit organization that ensures safety during scuba diving and prevents underwater injuries.

- Your son has febrile seizures.
- He has seizures exclusively during sleep, and the last seizure was more than 3 years ago.
- He has other provoked seizures—**convulsive syncope**, seizures due to glucose or other electrolytes imbalance, or low blood pressure.

convulsive syncope

A brief loss of consciousness (syncope) associated with mild convulsions and stiffening.

69. My daughter had her first seizure 2 days after the DPT shot. Should she have other immunizations or hold off?

Fever, encephalopathy, or seizures could rarely occur after immunization. The possibility of seizure is very low. Do not forget that the appearance of seizures could be just coincidental or associated with fever caused by vaccination. A vaccination may act as a trigger to unmask the underlying neurological disorder associated with seizure disorder. Possibly, the vaccination is in a true sense responsible for seizures—a causal relationship.

A vaccination may act as a trigger to unmask the underlying neurological disorder associated with seizure disorder.

The diphtheria, pertussis, and tetatnus (DPT) vaccine has long been associated with encephalopathy in different studies. It is the pertussis component that has been incriminated to cause encephalopathy. This is a controversial and poorly understood field. It is unkown what components of the pertussis vaccine could cause encephalopathy or neurological damage. There have been a few studies that tried to compare the incidence of febrile seizures after diphtheria and tetanus versus DPT shot to determine the association of pertussis and febrile seizures in humans. There is 2–3 times increased risk of seizures after the use of pertussis vaccine. However, a febrile seizure does not lead to chronic epilepsy. The measles, mumps, and rubella

(MMR) vaccination has been associated with a very slight and transient increase in the incidence of febrile seizures. The overall long-term rate of epilepsy is not increased in children who had febrile seizures after vaccination. There are no long-term sequelae of increased risk of seizures following the DPT or MMR vaccine. Neither vaccine is associated with afebrile seizures. Vaccines may trigger infantile spasms. We do not have much understanding about the association of neonatal seizures and vaccines. Children with epilepsy should be fully immunized.

70. I have a child with seizures. What are the chances of my other children acquiring epilepsy?

genetics

Relating to genes.

Genetics definitely has an influence on epilepsy. Sometimes epilepsy runs in families. Environmental factors do play a role as well. Childhood epilepsies may be genetically driven and tend to be earlier in onset, during childhood and adolescence. Specific genes are involved in the susceptibility of certain epilepsies. However, not all epilepsies are inherited. Epilepsies secondary to head trauma or brain infections, stroke, or tumor are due to brain insult and may have no genetic influence. Some epilepsy syndromes such as benign neonatal and benign infantile convulsions are age related, have a benign course, and are rare syndromes. Febrile seizures— seizures related to fever—have onset during infancy or early childhood. This is a perfect example of interplay between environment and genetics. There is a higher incidence of febrile seizures in children of adult patients with febrile seizures. The siblings and first-degree relatives carry a higher risk as well. Sometimes febrile seizures are associated with other seizure types such as myoclonic, absence, myoclonic-astatic, atonic, and generalized tonic-clonic seizures without fever. This is called **generalized epilepsy with febrile seizures plus (GEFS+)** and results from mutation in the sodium channel gene. Unlike febrile seizures, the seizures in GEFS+ can persist beyond early childhood up to 6 years of age.

Overall, genetics has a stronger influence on generalized epilepsies in comparison to partial epilepsies. Childhood absence and juvenile myoclonic epilepsy are two such generalized epilepsies. Some of the examples of partial epilepsies with genetic influence are benign rolandic epilepsy and partial temporal lobe epilepsy with auditory features. The genetics risk diminishes as people get older, and there is no definite genetic influence after 35 years of age. Epilepsy in children with known injuries to the brain is not so genetically driven. Examples are children with head trauma; brain tumors, strokes, brain infections, and cerebral palsy do not carry an increased risk of genetic transmission. The genes associated with epilepsy syndromes are expressed in a complex manner and have variable degrees of expression. The inheritance of a specific gene does not result in the disease, and therefore, all gene carriers are not affected. This phenomenon is called **reduced penetrance**. Therefore, it may be hard to establish a direct link between a gene and development of epilepsy. Multiple genes may be responsible for the emergence of epilepsy. The majority of the epilepsy genes discovered to date are responsible for making normal ion channels. These channels are important for normal functioning of the nerve cells. Sodium, potassium, calcium, and chloride channels are the key players in controlling the excitability of the nerve cell membranes. Better understanding of how

Miscellaneous

generalized epilepsy with febrile seizures plus (GEFS+)

An epilepsy syndrome with different seizure types such as tonic-clonic, myoclonic, absence, atonic, or febrile seizure.

reduced penetrance

The mutated gene effect is modified or reduced and does not always cause disease when present.

155

these channels work and are affected in various epilepsies would be extremely crucial to find treatment strategies and drug options to treat epilepsy or these channelopathies (diseases of the ion channels).

Table 36 depicts some of the genetically inherited epilepsy syndromes. For the majority of other forms of epilepsies, the genetic influence is still undetermined. Certain kinds of epilepsies are more influenced by our genetic makeup than others. There is an ongoing multicenter study trying to answer the same question as to how genetic factors play a part in causing epilepsy. The Epilepsy Phenome Genome Project study is funded by the National Institutes of Health and is a coordinated effort of more than fourteen epilepsy treatment sites. This project, when completed, could shed more light on some unanswered questions.

71. I am a would-be mother, but I have a seizure disorder. I am taking all these medications. Can these have deleterious effects on my baby?

The use of medications certainly increases the risk of birth defects. The increased frequency of seizures may

---

Table 36 Genetically Inherited Epilepsy Syndromes

- Benign infantile convulsions
- Benign neonatal convulsions
- Benign rolandic epilepsy
- Childhood absence epilepsy
- Generalized epilepsy with febrile seizures plus (GEFS+)
- Febrile seizures
- Juvenile absence epilepsy
- Juvenile myoclonic epilepsy
- Nocturnal frontal lobe epilepsy
- Partial epilepsy with auditory features

---

itself be responsible for birth defects. The risk differs for different medications. This risk is higher when one is taking several medications compared to someone else who is only on one medication. The risk increases if you are taking higher dosages of medications. You can reduce the risk of birth defects by taking folic acid on a regular basis. Folic acid is crucial to prevent some of the serious birth defects related to the brain and spinal cord. These are called neural tube defects. **Neural tube** is one of the key structures in the early development of the brain and spinal cord. The risk of neural tube defect is lower if you take folic acid before you get pregnant.

The birth defects can be minor or major. Major birth defects can affect skin, nails, or mucous membranes. Some examples are cleft lip or cleft palate, which can be surgically repaired once the child is born. Fortunately, the major birth defects are rare. Major birth defects include heart, kidneys, or neural tube defects. Most of the birth defects can be detected by doing ultrasound of the baby. Pregnant mothers can be tested for other markers in the blood plasma (serum) or amniotic fluid. One important marker is called **alpha-fetoprotein**. Alpha-fetoprotein screening has been available since the early 1980s. This is an important screening test for a subset of developmental abnormalities including neural tube defects. If the level of alpha-fetoprotein is abnormal, the prenatal ultrasound test is performed to look for fetal abnormalities. Another option is to measure the alpha-fetoprotein in the amniotic fluid by performing amniocentesis. Amniocentesis provides health and maturity status of the fetus and is used to obtain genetic information as well.

If you are pregnant and are currently taking medications, I would encourage you to enroll in the pregnancy registry. All women of childbearing age and on one or more

neural tube
A precursor of the central nervous system.

alpha-fetoprotein
An antigen present in the human fetus and in diseased conditions in the adult.

medications to treat seizures should enroll in the registry. The different registries try to study the adverse effects of antiepileptics on your baby. Your enrollment helps them to find answers to some of the questions you or your doctors may have regarding the safety of medications during pregnancy. Even though new medications are approved by the FDA, doctors and patients need to find out the safety of these new medications during pregnancy. The information provided by you is kept completely confidential. Your name is not indicated in the database. The information is filed in a database, but pharmaceutical companies, physicians, and the health insurance companies do not have access to this database. I would encourage you to enroll as early as possible. Most of the registries contact you during pregnancy and after your baby is born to see how you are doing.

72. Can I breast-feed my baby?

The benefits of breast-feeding outweigh the potential risk of exposure of a newborn to antiepileptics.

I would strongly encourage you to breast-feed your baby. The benefits of breast-feeding outweigh the potential risk of exposure of a newborn to antiepileptics. Mother's milk is important because it contains anti-infective factors that build up the immunity of your baby in the early months of infancy. It is easily digestible and protects your baby from several intestinal infections. It is a rich source of carnitine, which helps develop a healthy liver. Breast-fed children are found to have higher IQs than those who were not breast-fed. Breast-feeding also establishes an emotional bond with the mother.

There is no doubt that antepileptics do get excreted in breast milk. The amount of drug excretion in milk depends on how avidly the drug binds to plasma proteins in the mother. If the drug has a very high protein binding, then less drug is excreted in the newborn. This explains why some AEDs are excreted more than others. Phenytoin, divalproex sodium, and tiagabine have high protein binding and get excreted in breast milk in very low concentrations. Carbamazepine, phenobarbital, lamotrigine, topiramate, and zonisamide have low-to-moderate protein binding and low-to-moderate concentrations in breast milk. Drugs like levetiracetam and gabapentin with no protein binding have equivalent concentrations in the mother and in breast milk.

AEDs can have some central nervous system side effects in the newborns if the drug concentration becomes significant in breast milk. You should watch the newborn for symptoms such as excessive sleepiness, irritability, jitteriness, or inadequate weight gain. If you find the newborn baby sedated or irritable, you can supplement breast milk with bottle feedings.

73. I have seizures. I am afraid of taking care of an infant. What precautions can I take to ensure the safety of my child?

Some women with epilepsy and frequent seizures choose not to get pregnant because they have the same concern you do. Infant safety guidelines should be discussed to prevent any mishaps and injury to the newborn. Sleep deprivation is not uncommon for any woman taking care of a newborn; this may cause an increase in the frequency of seizures. Try to catch up with your sleep when your baby is taking a nap. You can also express your milk with the help of a breast pump and store it. Someone else can help you with the nighttime feedings. You should sit on the floor or in the middle of the bed when you are feeding the baby. Sit on a mat when you are trying to change the infant's clothes or diapers. Try not to hold your baby in your arms while preparing the bottle feedings—the child is safer in the crib or bassinet. The crib should be in the same room where you sleep. Transporting the baby in a stroller is better than using a baby crib or carrying him or her on your shoulder. Try to give your baby his or her bath when there is someone else in the house. If you are all by yourself, then try to give the baby a sponge bath sitting on the floor. A playpen can be used as a safe place for the baby.

The toddler needs a different kind of care. They are much more accident prone. Their surroundings should be made as childproof as possible in case the toddler is alone with a parent who has a seizure with impairment or loss of consciousness. The bathroom and kitchen doors need to be locked so that toddlers do not put something into their mouths. Exits and stairwells should also be blocked so that toddlers do not walk out of the house or fall down the stairs.

As children grow, they can be taught how to dial 911, ask for help from the neighbors, or call significant others in such emergencies. They should have all important phone numbers handy, such as near the phone or on a refrigerator, and they should know their home address.

74. It has been very hard for our family and my son to deal with accepting the diagnosis of seizures. He does not enjoy doing things he used to do before, and his sleeping habits and appetite have changed. What can I do?

depression
Chronic feelings of sadness, despair, and helplessness.

Epilepsy and psychiatric disorders are extremely common. The most common disorders are **depression, anx-**

iety, **psychosis**, and attention deficit/hyperactivity disorder. Depression is a **mood disorder** caused and carried on by an interaction of genetic, biological, psychological, and environmental factors. It has widespread effects on the mind and body, thoughts, feelings, behavior, and physical conditions. Symptoms generally vary.

Common symptoms are as follows:

- Irritability
- Loss of interest in activities
- Sadness
- Tiredness
- Anxiousness
- Feelings of worthlessness and hopelessness
- Argumentative behavior
- Aggression
- Wanting to be alone
- Headaches and stomachaches
- Problems eating and sleeping

The intensity and duration of symptoms of depression vary from person to person. Symptoms can lead to disruptive behavior, school problems, social problems, alcohol and drug use, fighting with siblings, and estranged relationships. Depression affects millions of people across socioeconomic lines. It can run in families. About 4% of teenagers are depressed; this figure is still on the rise.

Symptoms result from abnormality in the way the brain produces and maintains levels of chemicals that are involved in transmitting messages from nerve cell to nerve cell.

Normally, neurons in the brain and all over the body send electrical signals through **axons** (long, stemlike

anxiety
Excessive, ongoing worry and tension.

psychosis
A mental disorder in which delusions and hallucinations are combined.

mood disorder
Disturbance of mood such as major depression, mania, or hypomania.

axon
Part of a neuron that conducts impulses away from the cell body.

Miscellaneous

projections found on neurons); on the ends of axons are branchlike nerve endings that contain storage sacs, which release chemicals called neurotransmitters. Neurotransmitters carry the message across a tiny, fluid-filled gap called a synapse; on the next neuron are receptors which, when activated, cause the neuron to become activated. Depression breaks down this complex system, resulting in an inadequate amount of certain neurotransmitters present in the brain—abnormal amounts absorbed, destroyed, and/or released from nerve endings. Neurotransmitters, specifically norepinephrine and serotonin, are connected to depression. Norepinephrine and serotonin regulate mood and level of alertness. Inadequate concentration of neurotransmitters causes fatigue and sadness. Dopamine, another neurotransmitter, also affects mood (a higher level in the brain correlates with a more upbeat mood).

Depression in children with epilepsy can be multifactorial. It can be the result of psychosocial burdens of epilepsy when one is identified as different from a normal child. Psychiatric disorders may be present independent of epilepsy, perhaps as a result of the child's genetic makeup. There may be other family members with a history of depression, alcoholism, or bipolar disorder. At times it is hard to tease out clearly if these are the complications of medical or surgical treatment. The FDA issued new information on January 31, 2008 to alert physicians about the increased risk of suicidal thoughts and behaviors in patients treated with AEDs. The FDA's position is that all medications in the antiepileptic class share the increased risk of suicidality. The FDA recommends that families should be informed about these side effects and patients should be carefully observed for any behavioral changes.

Almost all drugs can result in behavioral problems. No matter what the etiology is, these are underrecognized, underdiagnosed, and underaddressed. Children may not even understand the symptoms of depression or mood disorders or may not feel comfortable discussing the symptoms with parents or their physicians. Patients try to minimize their psychiatric symptoms. Parents may not be forthcoming in telling the physicians that their child gets frustrated easily or has become more withdrawn and is not doing activities as before. The physicians may be focusing more on their seizure calendars and the optimal control in the short office visits and may completely fail to inquire about the psychiatric symptoms. The coexisting depression and anxiety can have a negative impact on the optimal control of seizures, as any kind of mental stress can exacerbate seizures. The coexisting psychiatric morbidities can affect sleep patterns. Inability to fall asleep at night or maintain sleep, and frequent arousals are commonly encountered problems. At times, it is hard to tease out whether symptoms such as weight gain, trouble sleeping, fragmented sleep, excessive daytime sleepiness, fatigue, or insomnia are the result of coexisting depression or the side effects of AEDs and psychiatric medications. Lack of proper sleep can provoke seizures. Poor performance at school, lower grades in the school report card, and teacher notes to parents that a child is not focusing on schoolwork may be other clues that something is wrong.

Depression and mood changes can be seen before, during, and after the seizures. The prevalence of depression is about 20–55% in patients with recurrent seizures. The prevalence is as low as 3–9% in patients with well-controlled seizures. Some patients are not able to define their auras, but parents can tell their child behaves differently, hours or days before a seizure.

After seizures, children may experience hopelessness, frustration, helplessness, low self-esteem, irritability, guilt, or self-deprecation. I have had parents reporting to me that their child is a different person and can have disordered thought at times after a cluster of seizures. This is called **postictal psychosis** and is seen within 1 week of a seizure or cluster of seizures. These symptoms can last at least 15 hours but should not last more than 2 months. It is important to exclude psychoses caused by drugs or other preexisting psychiatric conditions. Patients with head injury and brain infections are more likely to have postictal psychosis.

postictal psychosis

A state of psychosis occurring after a seizure. *See* psychosis.

It is incumbent on the physician to find some time to think beyond seizure control and find out about a child's behavior at school and his or her academic performance. Depression should be treated with psychotherapy and antidepressants. A lot of patients ask whether the use of antidepressants is safe with antiepileptics. Antidepressants should be carefully selected, as few antidepressants can lower seizure threshold or lower the metabolism of the AEDs causing higher blood levels. For example, bupropion is a great antidepressant, but when used at higher dosages of more than 300 mg/day, it can lower the seizure threshold. Fluvoxamine (Luvox), fluoxetine (Prozac), and paroxetine (Paxil) can have drug interactions with AEDs and increase the concentrations of AEDs. Experience with cilatopram (Celexa), escitalopram (Lexapro), venlafaxine (Effexor), and sertraline (Zoloft) has been very positive, and their use as antidepressants has been considered safe in patients with epilepsy.

At times, it is hard to differentiate whether mood swings are just normal teenage behavior or the effects of seizures or medications.

Bizarre behavior can be of paramount significance for some children with epilepsy and their families. The physician may find it challenging to control behavior versus seizures. The children can have an excellent control of seizures for a short time but the behavior can be totally out of control or vice versa. This is called **forced normalization**. On the other hand, injudicial use of drugs can lower the seizure threshold. It is prudent that your physician has a thorough understanding of the drug-to-drug interactions between antidepressants, antianxiety drugs, and antiepileptics.

Bizarre behavior can be of paramount significance for some children with epilepsy and their families.

forced normalization

A relationship between seizure control and psychotic symptoms that exists in some patients with intractable epilepsies.

Miscellaneous

75. My son has been getting attacks of blurred vision, nausea, and vomiting. These symptoms are followed by a bad headache. I am concerned that these could be signs of a brain tumor. Can these be seizures?

After taking a detailed history about these episodes, I suspect these are migraine headaches. His neurological examination is completely normal. I do not think he needs an MRI or CAT scan at this time. A typical migraine attack is described as throbbing headache, as it involves blood vessels in the brain. People fear this to be arising from brain tumor because it is intense and pulsating in nature. Pain is on both sides of the temples or the forehead regions. In adults it could be on one side or the other, and the sides could alternate. Symptoms of nausea and vomiting are common in young children. There are known triggers of migraines such as sleep deprivation, chocolate, red wine, processed meats, monosodium glutamate, aged cheese, and too much caffeine. Recurrent symptoms of migraines are confused with seizures especially if there is loss of consciousness. Migraines are common in patients with epilepsy. This close association is well recognized. **Migralepsy** is the term used when a seizure occurs during or within 1 hour of a typical migraine attack. Up to one-quarter of patients with epilepsy have a history of migraines. Migraine is at least 2.4 times higher in patients with epilepsy compared to others without epilepsy. Migraine is equally common in boys and girls before puberty. In the postpubertal period, it is much more common in females. Migraines run in families. It is not uncommon to find several family members or relatives suffering from the same condition.

Migraines can be with or without aura. Patients often experience visual symptoms described as their aura. However, it is uncommon to have an aura in children younger than 8 years of age. Migraines tend to be shorter in duration, less than 4 hours in children. About two-thirds of children do not experience an aura. Children can be very sensitive to light or sounds. These are referred to as **photophobia** and **phonophobia**, respectively. Pain may be triggered by movement and relieved by sleeping in a quiet, dark room. There are different migraine types in children.

Migraine with aura (classic migraine) presents with visual auras lasting 5–30 minutes followed by severe headaches. Your son may complain of zigzag lines, sparkling lights, or black and gray spots in front of his eyes. These are referred to as halos or scintillating scotomas. Scotoma is an area of lost or decreased vision

migralepsy

An old term that signifies the common association between epilepsy and migraine. It is used in the clinical context when a seizure occurs within one hour after a typical migraine attack with an aura.

photophobia

An abnormal or irrational fear of light.

phonophobia

Fear of sounds and noise.

migraine with aura (classic migraine)

Aura characterized by visual changes, nausea, vomiting, and trouble with light and sounds; followed by throbbing headache, pulsating in nature, lasting 4–72 hours.

within the visual field surrounded by an area of less depressed or normal vision. Other visual complaints include blurring of vision, complete loss of vision, or perceived changes in the size of objects. Migraine with aura is more closely tied to unprovoked seizures in children. The increased risk was found up to 3.7 times in various studies.

Migraine without aura (common migraine) is the most common migraine and lasts a few hours only. A prolonged attack lasting up to 72 hours is referred to as **status migrainosus**.

Complicated migraine is characterized by complex neurological symptoms and signs such as loss of motor and sensory functions or complete loss of vision. One half of the visual field on one or both eyes may be affected. This is called **hemianopia**. Cranial nerves may be involved. There are twelve cranial nerves in the brain, designated by roman numerals. The III cranial nerve, which supplies the eye, is typically involved in migraines. These deficits are transient but raise concerns about the nature of attacks. At times, it raises concerns about the possibility of a brain tumor in the occipital area or temporal or **parietal lobe**. The presence of colored halos also raises the concerns of tumor in the occipital area. The prolonged attacks of migraine may be associated with mild abnormalities on the MRI of the brain.

Basilar migraine can be associated with loss of consciousness. This state of altered consciousness raises concerns about complex partial seizures, as patients usually get bad headaches after seizures. This is the most common migraine variant in children. Patients with

Miscellaneous

migraine without aura (common migraine)

The most common form of migraine in which a patient has recurring headaches lasting 4–12 hours. Headaches are not preceded by an aura and tend to be unilateral, pulsating in quality, with nausea and/or vomiting, and trouble with lights or sounds.

status migrainosus

A rare, continuous, prolonged, intense, and unremitting migraine attack lasting longer than 72 hours.

complicated migraine

Migraines associated with complex neurological symptoms such as weakness, loss of sensations, or visual or speech problems.

hemianopia

Blindness in one half of the visual field of one or both eyes.

parietal lobe

The part of the brain that is involved in perceiving sensations.

basilar migraine

A migraine associated with complicated symptoms such as slurred speech, loss of balance, or brief loss of consciousness.

basilar migraine experience brain stem symptoms. The brain stem is the lower part of the brain. Common brain stem symptoms include double vision, dizziness, loss of balance sensation, ringing in the ears, slurred speech, or a true vertigo. Vertigo is an illusion of spinning movements. Patients describe this as "the room is spinning" or they are spinning in relation to their surroundings. Alteration in the level of consciousness may result from involvement of the reticular activating system. The reticular activating system is believed to be the center of arousal and is crucial for maintaining the state of consciousness.

Cyclic vomiting is characterized by repeated episodes of severe vomiting lasting from hours to days. In between the attacks, the child is completely normal. It is more common in white children and has a slight female preponderance. Many patients with cyclic vomiting have symptoms resembling those of migraines such as headaches, nausea, vomiting, and trouble with lights or sounds, and they respond well to antimigraine treatments.

Confusional migraine is characterized by periods of confusion and disorientation lasting 4–6 hours followed by deep sleep. Children do not complain of headache but appear very uncomfortable, irritable, and confused. Confusional migraine is misdiagnosed as complex partial seizures. A careful history can tease out the difference and avoid wrong treatment.

Migraine aura without headache can occur. This is called **acephalgic migraine**.

Alternating hemiplegia of childhood is a childhood disorder presenting before 18 months of age and is char-

cyclic vomiting

Considered a kind of migraine disorder seen more commonly in children between 3–7 years of age and characterized by bouts or cycles of severe nausea or vomiting that last for hours or even days.

confusional migraine

A type of migraine seen in children that causes a confusional state characterized by inattention and difficulty with speech and motor activities.

acephalgic migraine

Symptoms such as visual changes, nausea, and vomiting experienced by a migraineur; these are not followed by headaches.

alternating hemiplegic migraine (AHC)

A type of migraine that is characterized by vomiting, headache, loss of consciousness, and alternating paralysis/weakness of the body. It is a disease of childhood that sets in before age 18 months.

acterized by weakness of one side or the other alternating from one side to the other.

Headaches can occur after seizures as well. This is called postictal headache. Some patients complain of headache before their seizures.

76. *What are early intervention programs?*

Children differ in their intellect and physical development. Children with special needs should be recognized early on and carefully placed in the right environment conducive to their physical, psychosocial, and emotional needs. Early help does make a difference! The mental development is most rapid in the first 6 years of life. The child's improved mental and physical developmental reaps economic gains to the individual, family, and society, and minimizes dependence on assistance programs in the future. **Early intervention programs** offer a plethora of services such as educational meetings and symposia, support groups, and counseling. Early intervention programs go a long way to help children less than 3 years of age and should be provided to infants and toddlers with developmental delays and learning disabilities. These services are not limited to physical, occupational, or speech therapy but encompass their nutritional, nursing, and social needs. Provisions are made to meet their special sensory needs, such as vision and hearing, and other assistive devices can improve their speech, ambulation, or motor coordination. Transportation services may also be available. You can acquire more information about these programs by contacting a municipal early intervention official locally. These programs can help with developmental assessment of your

early intervention program (EIP)

A statewide program, run by Department of Health, which provides several services to infants and toddlers to promote physical, mental, and social development.

Miscellaneous

child and enrollment of kids for intervention programs without any cost to you.

77. What is ABA therapy?

Applied behavior analysis (ABA) is a practice to learn skills about learning. Children with autism, mental illness, developmental disabilities, and learning disorders get benefits from ABA; they learn how to talk, play, and live in a society. ABA is about providing autistic kids a structured environment where kids can learn as soon as possible. Interventionists such as parents, staff, and teachers help reinforce appropriate behaviors in different settings such as homes, schools, institutions, or group homes. Special emphasis is placed on language, social, academic, and functional life skills. Children are also taught to reduce self-injurious and stereotypic behaviors. Discrete trial teaching and natural environment training are different important approaches used for ABA therapy.

78. When I saw my son having a seizure, I wondered if he would die. Can you die during a seizure?

The risk of sudden unexplained death in children is very low. The risk of SUDEP (Sudden unexplained death in epilepsy) with ongoing seizures is better studied in children. Children with symptomatic generalized epilepsy with nighttime tonic-clonic seizures are more prone to SUDEP. SUDEP can also occur after a complex partial seizure. Boys may be more vulnerable than girls. Children and adolescents with poorly controlled seizures who are placed on multiple medications carry a higher risk. Frequent changes in medications, low drug levels, and poor adherence to medical treatment have been incriminated in SUDEP cases. Physicians have to use their judgment and discretion as to when to inform the parents and families about SUDEP. Inadequate patient instructions or education, intolerable side effects of medications, and complex dosing scheduling could be some of the causes of nonadherence to treatment. However, an open and honest dialogue between the families and physician is important to achieve adequate seizure control or remission without adverse side effects. Parents should be informed that children or adolescents with infrequent seizures are not immune to SUDEP.

PART SEVEN

Epilepsy Surgery

Is epilepsy surgery an option for children?

What are the benefits and risks of surgery?

Is my child a good surgical candidate?
How do you determine that?

More ...

79. Is epilepsy surgery an option for children?

Epilepsy surgery is an option in selected cases when children have frequent intractable seizures and medications not only fail to control seizures but in addition cause tolerance issues or side effects. The timing of surgical intervention is crucial because the child's nervous system has **neuroplasticity**. A child's brain can facilitate reorganization of cortical networks more flexibly than an adult brain. Several factors, listed next, need to be considered while making surgical decisions:

neuroplasticity

Reorganization of brain networks and ability to regenerate to a limited extent.

- Ongoing seizures and their cognitive and behavioral impact
- Tolerability of medications
- Quality of life and lifestyle limitations
- Seizure foci—single or multiple
- Seizure types
- Safety of surgery based on presurgical testing

With the advent of sophisticated neurosurgical techniques, surgery is being considered more often and earlier in children. Presurgical testing can help determine the risks and benefits of the surgery. Surgery has a better outcome when there is a structural abnormality in the brain, such as scar tissue from the temporal lobe in temporal lobe epilepsy; an abnormal vascular malformation, such as a **cavernoma**, a low-grade or high-grade tumor causing compression of the neighboring areas of the brain and intractable seizures; an abnormal collection of neurons as a result of migrational defect, such as a tuber in patients with tuberous sclerosis; or any other cortical dysplasia. Children with structural lesions have a visualized target seen on the MRI that can be tackled with least invasive neurosurgical techniques minimizing postoperative deficits.

cavernoma

One type of malformation of the blood vessels in the brain. It can cause seizures, stroke symptoms, hemorrhages, and headache. It occurs relatively frequently in children.

80. What are the benefits and risks of surgery?

The seizure freedom after surgery can range from 40% to 100%. The chances of seizure freedom with medical therapy can be as low as 5% after two medications have failed. Surgery may not be curative in all patients, and not all patients are good surgical candidates. However, the success rates for epilepsy surgery are constantly improving as the technology is advancing and more noninvasive tests and radiologic techniques are available. A perfect case scenario would be to be seizure free and medication free after the epilepsy surgery. Some patients may still need to continue their medications at the same or reduced dosages. Reduced seizure burden and less medications in the long run make surgery still worth considering in very complicated cases. Corpus callosotomy can be helpful in preventing head injuries. Vagal nerve stimulator not only reduces seizure frequency but also helps symptoms of depression and anxiety, improving overall quality of life.

Permanent complications associated with surgery are very low. The risk of death is low, from 0.1% to 1%. However, general anesthesia itself carries a risk of death. Surgery carries increased risk of complications in young infants from 0 to 5 months. Other risks include bleeding in the brain or infection or bone resorption, but risk is less than 1%. Hydrocephalus (increased fluid in the brain) can develop due to obstruction in the flow of cerebrospinal fluid. Brain surgery always has the potential of causing additional neurological deficits, stroke, or paralysis. Stroke can cause motor or sensory deficits and thought and language difficulties. Mild peripheral vision loss, third cranial nerve palsy, memory and language difficulties, and mood changes may be seen with temporal lobe surgery. There is always a remote but rare possibility that seizures will get worse after epilepsy surgery. Neuropsychologic testing is done preoperatively and 6 months to 1 year after the surgery. Children have more plasticity to counteract any memory deficits after the surgery compared to adults. See **Table 37** for help with minor memory problems.

81. Is my child a good surgical candidate? How do you determine that?

Your child's epileptologist or neurologist runs a gamut of tests on her to determine the safety of surgery. These are called presurgical tests. The extent of presurgical testing is determined on an individual basis. A few epilepsy surgeries are straightforward and do not require all the tests discussed herein. It is important to predetermine whether the area of the brain the surgeon is planning to remove is the actual source of the seizures. These tests include:

- History
- Neurolgic examination
- MRI of the brain
- EEG
- Video EEG

Table 37 Ways to Combat Memory Deficits	
External	**Internal**
Wall hooks for keys, placing items by the door, special shelves, filing systems	Outlining techniques
	Mnemonics
Notebook/diary	Alarms as reminders
Calendar	Pagers
Checklist systems	
PDA	
Sticky notes	
To-do lists	

- Neuropsychological testing
- Wada testing
- PET
- SPECT
- MRS
- MEG

The results of the aforementioned tests are discussed in a multidisciplinary surgical conference in great detail. The multidisciplinary conference is attended by pediatric neurologists, epileptologists, **neurosurgeons**, neuropsychologists, nurse practitioners, and paramedical staff. Physicians discuss your child's history, neurological examination findings, and results of diagnostic tests to determine how safe the surgery is. What is the impact of seizures on your developing child's brain? What are the risks involved in removing the seizure focus? What are the chances of seizure freedom? If all test results line up well, your child stands a good chance of seizure freedom. Surgical outcome may be less favorable if test results do not line up well, if there are multiple seizure foci, or if seizure focus cannot be completely removed because of risk of losing some important function of the brain.

82. We were told by the other epilepsy center that a burr-hole operation or survey study can better define the seizure focus. What is a survey study?

In a survey study, small openings called **burr holes** are made in the skull bone with a surgical drill. Strip electrodes (shown in **Figure 15a**) are inserted under the covering of the brain called dura (**Figure15b**). Strip

Epilepsy Surgery

neurosurgeon
Surgeon who carries out surgery for the treatment of conditions of the nervous system.

burr hole
A small opening in the skull made with a surgical drill.

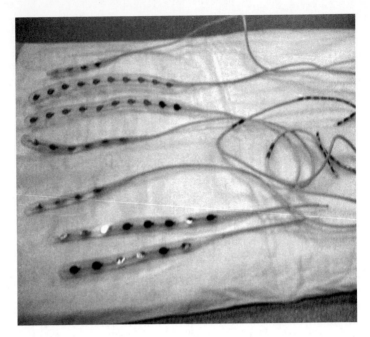

Figure 15a
Strip electrodes. *Source:* Reproduced from Singh A. 2006. *100 Questions and Answers About Epilepsy.* Sudbury, Massachusetts: Jones and Bartlett Publishers, LLC.

electrodes covering both hemispheres determine if seizures start from the left or right side of the brain. This is also referred to as a survey study. Frontal and temporal areas of the brain are studied the most, but parietal and **occipital lobes** can be covered as well. There is a small risk of infection with the placement of subdural electrodes. The infection can occur in 1–3% of patients. Judicious use of antibiotics can reduce the risk of infection.

Scalp EEG has its own limitations. The electrodes used to monitor EEG activity are far away from the brain. There is intervening skin, muscle, bone, cerebrospinal fluid between the brain, and electrodes. At times the seizure onset is obscured by muscle and movement arti-

occipital lobe
The part of the brain that plays a part in visual perception.

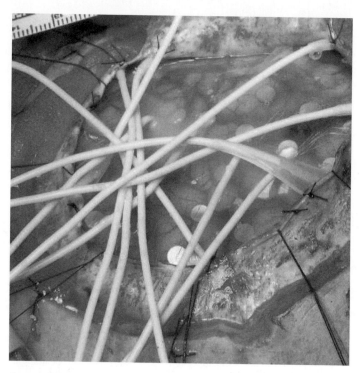

Figure 15b
Bilateral subdural strips.

fact. Seizures clinically may look the same suggesting a single focus, but it is hard for the clinicians to tell if it started from the right hemisphere or the left. One such example is frontal lobe partial seizures. Patients may have thrashing movements in frontal seizures causing a lot of muscle and movement artifact. Seizures may be brief, causing failure to show sustained changes on the EEG. Frontal seizures spread to the other hemisphere very quickly and may show no focal changes on one side of the brain.

Another example of when a bilateral survey study could be helpful is tuberous sclerosis. The majority of seizures may be coming from one focus even if someone has multiple foci. A bilateral survey study can be helpful in such circumstances.

83. What is brain mapping? Is it painful?

Brain mapping is done to map out the functional areas of the brain. Different areas of the brain have designated functions. Brain mapping delineates these vital functions and makes a road map for the neurosurgeon. During brain mapping, the brain is stimulated to know the specific functional areas of the brain, and seizure focus is mapped (see **Figure 16a**). Brain mapping is done after

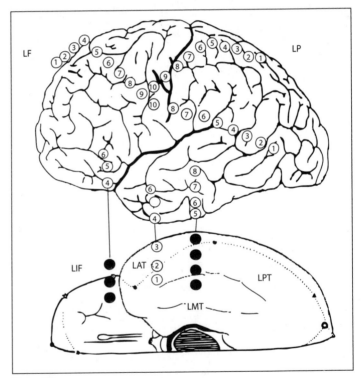

Figure 16a
Seizure foci on intracranial mapping. Black circles on different electrode points on the strips depict different seizure foci. *Source:* Reproduced from Singh A. 2006. *100 Questions and Answers About Epilepsy.* Sudbury, Massachusetts: Jones and Bartlett Publishers, LLC.

grids, strips, or depths have been implanted. Mapping can be done in the epilepsy monitoring unit by the bedside. It can also be performed in the operating room while the patient is awake. It is not a painful procedure. However, there is a relatively small risk of pain during electrical stimulation. The brain itself does not sense the currents, but occasionally an electrode can make contact with the membranes surrounding the brain. Stimulation at these sites with higher currents can help avoid the discomfort.

Motor and language mapping are the most commonly performed mappings. **Figure 16b** depicts mapped language areas of the brain with black circles. Sensory and visual functions can also be mapped. It usually takes 1.5–2 hours to perform this test. The time required to perform brain mapping varies depending upon how many regions of the brain need to be tested and what

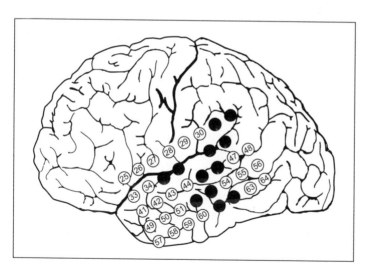

Figure 16b
Language mapping of the brain. Black circles on the grid signify language centers of the brain. *Source:* Reproduced from Singh A. 2006. *100 Questions and Answers About Epilepsy.* Sudbury, Massachusetts: Jones and Bartlett Publishers, LLC.

kind of function is expected from those areas. Brain mapping requires cooperation from the patient and may not be feasible in very young children. The procedure can last longer if the patient is uncooperative. Brain mapping is done in the EMU once your child's epileptologist has captured a sufficient number of seizures and has a **seizure map** based on **intracranial recordings**. The patient is placed back on medications and may even be loaded with AEDs to minimize the risk of seizures during the procedure.

A very low current is applied to a very small area of the brain. This brief stimulation of current interrupts the normal functioning of the brain. For example, a speech arrest can be observed if language areas are stimulated. Mouth movements may be seen if areas controlling mouth movements are stimulated. The function returns to its normal state once the stimulus is withdrawn. The epileptologist starts with the lowest possible current and increases the current until a significant response is reached. During mapping, negative and positive phenomena are carefully assessed. Negative phenomena include weakness, numbness of an arm or leg, or facial droop. Examples of positive phenomena are jaw protrusion, twitching, electric feeling, or tingling in the face, arm, or leg. At times, seizures may be triggered by stimulation of the brain if the epileptologist is near the seizure focus. This may interrupt the procedure but gives valuable information to the team. Electrical stimulation can be interrupted as soon as these discharges build up. A functional map and a seizure map give valuable information to the neurosurgeon. It helps navigating during brain surgery. It provides guidance as to what areas are involved in the seizure and should be taken out, and what areas have important functions and should be avoided.

seizure map

A map of the brain indicating in what part of the brain seizure seems to be originating.

intracranial recording

EEG recording from intracranial electrodes (electrode grid/strips placed directly on the cortical surface or implanted depth electrode).

A functional map and a seizure map give valuable information to the neurosurgeon.

84. What is Wada testing?

Wada is an important presurgical test done before some epilepsy surgeries. It is also known by another name, the **intracarotid sodium amobarbital test**. Wada is named after Dr. Juhn Atsushi Wada, a Japanese-Canadian neurosurgeon who invented this test. The brain has two sides called hemispheres—right and left. The left hemisphere is a predominant language center in about 96% of all right-handed individuals and 70% of left-handers. Left-handers and ambidextrous (no predominance of handedness) individuals have bilateral language presentation in 15% of cases and right hemisphere language predominance in another 15%.

The first part of the test requires a **cerebral angiogram** (study of the blood vessels of the brain), which is performed by intervention **neuroradiologists**. **Neurointerventional radiology** is a special medical field dedicated to the treatment of vascular diseases of the central nervous system. A catheter is passed into a femoral artery in the groin under local anesthesia. The catheter is then directed toward the right and left internal carotid artery. Carotid arteries are the major blood vessels supplying the brain. The images of blood vessels of the brain are taken, and any abnormalities in the vessels supplying the brain are determined at this time. A dye called **sodium amobarbital** is then injected into each carotid artery alternately. This dye puts half of the brain to sleep. The two injections are referred to as first injection and second injection. The injected side of the brain goes to sleep, or behaves like an artificially induced state of paralysis or stroke of half of the brain. The effects of the dye are transient and wear off in 10–20 minutes. The dose administered is 80–120 mg. Patients may complain of warm sensation as the dye is injected. Some

Wada

A frequently performed presurgical test before epilepsy surgery. It is also called a language-memory test.

intracarotid sodium amobarbital test

Also called Wada test, used to localize speech and memory function prior to epilepsy surgery.

cerebral angiogram

An X-ray of the arteries and veins in the brain.

neuroradiologist

Specialist who uses imaging devices and substances to study the brain.

neurointerventional radiology

A specialized branch of radiology that helps diagnosing and treating disorders of the blood vessels of the head, spine, and neck.

sodium amobarbital

A barbiturate drug that is injected into one hemisphere of the brain and shuts down the functions of language, motor, and memory in that hemisphere.

Epilepsy Surgery

patients get drowsy with the higher dose. The diseased side is always studied first. If the doctors feel that the seizure focus is on the right side, they put the left side of the brain to sleep first and study the language and memory functions of the right side of the brain.

A team of epileptologists examines the patient after the dye is injected and tries to determine whether the optimal dose is given, causing the transient paralysis of half of the brain. As the injection is given, the patient is asked to hold his or her arms up in the air and count aloud 1, 2, 3, etc. The optimal dose of the drug is determined by judging the strength in the arms. As the optimal level of the drug reaches the brain, the patient is not able to hold one of his or her arms in the air and drops it. If the injected side of the brain has important language functions, the patient is not able to count aloud. After the first injection and during the maximal dose effect, the team of neuropsychologists assesses the language and memory functions in details. The Wada evaluation is another way to lateralize language as well as memory functions. This test allows the neuropsychologist to independently test the cognitive function of a cerebral hemisphere while the other hemisphere is asleep. Language is assessed in different ways—comprehension, ability to speak or repeat or name different visual stimuli (drawings, printed words, colored shapes, or simple arithmetic problems), body parts, or common objects. Different pictures or objects are shown to the patient. The number of items shown to the patient varies from institution to institution. The patient is asked to name the objects. The patient may not be able to name the objects or be able to repeat the verbal commands if his or her language ability is affected, but the patient looks at the pictures and is asked to remember them. The patient's language and memory scores are charted by the neuropsychologists. The score is charted as a ratio. The denominator reflects the number of items shown. The numerator is the patient's score. A score of 0/12 reflects a very poor memory and means that the patient was shown 12 items and did not remember any item. A score of 12/12 means a perfect score and means that he or she remembered all objects. It is believed that the diseased side or the side with a seizure focus should have a poor memory but that may not always be the case. Based on the patient's scores, the epileptologist, neuropsychologist, and neurosurgeon want to determine whether he or she is at risk of language or memory deficit if surgery is performed on a particular hemisphere. A very good score may increase the risk of memory or language deficits after the surgery. A very poor score may not be concerning and minimizes the postoperative risks of deficits. Wada allows the team to better plan surgical interventions, as this procedure provides valuable information about what type of cognitive changes, if any, may be expected if surgery is undertaken.

85. What could be the complications of Wada?

The Wada test is a safe procedure. However, it is invasive. There could always be complications, as major vessels are catheterized. Complications can be as minor as pain at the site of the catheter. Bleeding at the site can occur. Infection at the catheter site is possible but rare because of aseptic precautions. Serious complications such as a stroke are rare but possible. Stroke occurs when a small piece of fat inside an artery becomes loose and causes blockage of vessels in the brain. This risk of stroke is less than 1% and is more likely in the older population because hardening of vessels with cholesterol deposits (atherosclerosis) is more common in adults.

86. What is surgical treatment of status epilepticus?

Most of the epilepsy surgeries being performed are done as elective procedures. However, emergency surgery is an option for children with status epilepticus. Hemispherectomy is the standard of care for the treatment of refractory status epilepticus for Rasmussen's encephalitis. However, more focal resections can be done if the patient is in convulsive or nonconvulsive partial status. Focal, lobar (one lobe), and multilobar (multiple lobes) resections have been done successfully to treat partial status epilepticus. Corpus callosotomy, multiple pial resections, vagal nerve stimulator, and low-frequency repetitive cortical electrical stimulation are other options.

87. What is the role of early surgical intervention in children?

Brodie and Kwan studies in 2000 followed 525 patients from 9–93 years of age with new-onset epilepsy. They found that only in 44% of patients did the first drug work. The second drug or third drug worked as monotherapy in only 17% and 3%, respectively. This study revolutionized the whole approach of treating intractable epilepsy. In 20–30% of medically refractory patients, surgical options should be considered. Berg followed 613 children with newly diagnosed epilepsy and found 10% were intractable. Berg defined intractability as failure of two or more antiepileptics. The timing of epilepsy surgery in children is very crucial. Once two or three medicines fail to control seizures, it becomes incumbent on the part of the physician to make parents aware of the role of surgery in epilepsy patients.

There is enough evidence from studies in children that there are some forms of epilepsies that can result in progressive cognitive impairment. There is a risk of sudden, unexplained death with tonic-clonic seizures. In addition, there are concerns about the long-term consequences of use of anticonvulsants. Children's brains have more plasticity than those of adults. Parents may be very skeptical about the brain surgery because medical therapy has fewer risks and less permanent consequences. With some patients, it becomes clear early on that surgery is a reasonable option to control seizures. Patients with abnormal MRI of the brain or a structural abnormality such as brain tumor or abnormal blood vessels, or those with abnormal migrational disorder can be excellent surgical candidates. A surgical approach is controversial for low-grade brain tumors. Patients with high-grade tumors require early intervention. These patients may need additional chemotherapy and radiation therapy. Patients with temporal lobe surgery and hippocampal sclerosis can be excellent surgical candidates.

88. When can our son return to school after the surgery?

It all depends on what surgical approach is being considered for your child. If your child is having a single-stage surgery, the stay in the hospital could be as short as 4–5 days. A two- or three-stage intracranial procedure takes longer. The average length of stay in the hospital is 7–14 days but may take longer, depending on how quickly seizures are captured between different stages of surgeries. Seizures may happen spontaneously or may require tapering of medications. The average recovery time from day one to release from the hospital to recuperation from the surgery is around 4–6 weeks. The recovery period may get extended if complications occur during surgery. Insertion of a vagal nerve stimulator is an outpatient procedure. Your child may have to miss 1–2 days of school, as the incision site could be painful.

89. What is a vagal nerve stimulator?

A vagal nerve stimulator (VNS) is a stimulation device, manufactured by Cyberonics, used to control seizures. This device is an FDA-approved minor epilepsy surgical tool. The exact mechanism of action of a VNS is unknown. It is believed that this device causes desynchronization of neuronal discharges to abort seizures. VNS has a pacemaker, a bipolar lead, and a programming wand with compatible computer/PDA and a handheld magnet **(Figures 17a and 17b)**. The pacemaker is made of titanium and does not generate any allergic reaction. The left vagal nerve has rich connections to the brain. The bipolar lead is tied around the vagal nerve fibers in the neck. The pacemaker is implanted subcutaneously somewhere below the clavicle. The right vagus is not attached because it has rich innervations to the heart and its stimulation can have deleterious effects on the heart. **Figure 18** shows positioning of various components of the VNS.

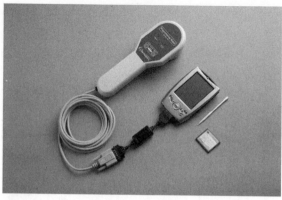

Figure 17a
Programming wand and PDA. *Source:* Copyright Cyberonics.

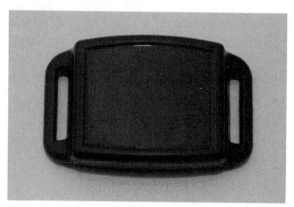

Figure 17b
Patient magnet. *Source:* Copyright Cyberonics.

The advantage of VNS is that there are not any side effects on the liver, brain, blood counts, bones, and other parts of the body.

VNS surgery is done in patients with multiple seizure foci. It is a reasonable option for those who continue to have seizures despite being on multiple medications or being unable to tolerate the medications' side effects. The advantage of VNS is that there are not any side effects on the liver, brain, blood counts, bones, and other parts of the body. Several studies have shown that decrease in mean seizure frequency by 40–50% in chil-

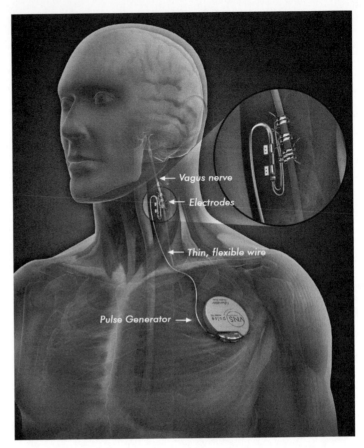

Figure 18
Positioning of implantable components. *Source:* Copyright Cyberonics.

dren more than 12 years of age. One does not have to worry about drug-to-drug interaction. VNS has been shown to have positive effects on mood and behavior and also improves quality of life measured by different parameters. A decrease in the frequency of seizures with VNS allows physicians to decrease medications. Another advantage is this surgery is minimally invasive, can be done as an outpatient, and gives families and patients a sense of control to a certain extent. It is a reversible outpatient procedure.

90. How long will it take to implant the VNS? What would be the cost of the device?

The surgery takes about 1–2 hours and is usually done as an outpatient procedure. The patient can be kept for observation only for a few hours. The procedure can be done under local or general anesthesia. Younger children often require general anesthesia. Two incisions are made, one in the chest wall below the collarbone or the armpit and the other in the neck to access the left vagus. The neurosurgeon makes a surgical pocket to implant a pulse generator under the skin of the patient's chest wall. The surgeon then threads a plastic tube containing the electrodes from the neck to the generator in the chest. The silicone-coated electrodes are then wrapped around the vagus nerve. Surgical complications are rare and include infection, wire lead erosion through the skin, or vocal cord paralysis.

VNS costs about $26,500. This includes the cost of the device and the surgery. Most of the insurance companies cover the cost. The manufacturing company Cyberonics also provides special assistance to families with inadequate medical coverage.

91. Would my daughter experience any side effects of the VNS? How often do I have to bring her for follow-up appointments after the VNS insertion?

VNS is well tolerated and has several advantages. This does not make your child sleepy, tired, and dizzy, unlike being on different AEDs. It does not have side effects on the liver or negative impact on your child's bone health. Patients and caretakers get a sense of control to a certain extent as they can swipe a magnet during a seizure. The device will send electrical signals to your daughter's brain at fixed intervals, but she will not feel the current. Studies have demonstrated positive effects on the level of alertness, verbal skills, mood, and memory. Patients have been able to reduce the number or dosages of medications after the VNS therapy. The VNS device does have mild common side effects as listed in **Table 38**.

The stimulation settings have to be programmed in a computer. Some epilepsy centers start the stimulation immediately after the surgery. Other centers wait until the next office visit. A typical parameter setting is 30 seconds on and 5 minutes off. The parameters are set with the help of a computer or a PDA device, special software, and a programming wand. Initially, patients might need programming every 2 weeks. Program adjustments take only few minutes and are tolerated well. The physician or the trained nurse uses a programming wand that converts the digital output from a personal computer to the radio frequency required for communication with the pulse generator and vice versa. The wand receives and sends signals to the personal computer via a cable connected to the wand by a phone

Table 38 Side Effects of Vagal Nerve Stimulators
Sore, painful throat
Shortness of breath
Heart rate and rhythm changes
Dizziness
Choking sensation
Difficulty swallowing
Facial flushing
Hiccuping
Left vocal cord paralysis
Hoarseness of voice

plug and to the computer by a standard serial connector. The medical staff opposes the wand to the center of the pulse generator.

Occasionally, a patient may cough or get hoarseness of voice as the settings are changed. The device can be turned off during eating to avoid swallowing problems. Patients who have underlying swallowing difficulties may experience worsening after the insertion of a VNS device. Some patients may turn the VNS off during public speaking to avoid hoarseness of voice. The VNS device, its parameters, and the battery life have to be checked at least every 6 months. The battery life depends on the device parameters—how often the electrical signals go to the brain. Patients whose VNS device is set on higher stimulation intensity and rapid cycling may use up the battery quickly. The battery life depends on the model used. With new models, the battery can last from 5–10 years (see **Table 39**). The new models are smaller and lighter in weight than the old models **(Figures 19a, b,** and **c)**.

Your daughter's physician may swipe the magnet to test if the battery is working properly. The new battery can be placed under local anesthesia. Parents have to understand that it is a reversible procedure. It is definitely not

Table 39 Various VNS Models and Their Approximate Battery Lives

Model	Approximate battery life
Model 100 (version B)	4–5 years
Model 100 (version C)	6–7 years
Model 101	9–10 years
Model 102	3–8 years
Model 102R	3–8 years
Model 103	3–8 years

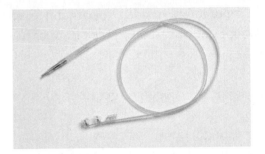

a.

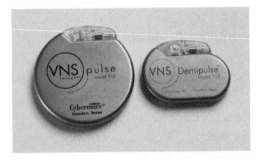

b.

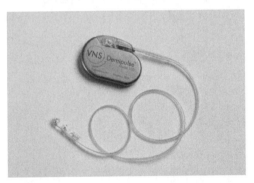

c.

Figure 19
Different models of VNS device: (a) 303 lead, (b) 102 and 103 demipulse generators, (c) 103 generator with 303 lead.
Source: Copyright Cyberonics.

a cure, but it has been effective in reducing the number of seizures and improves quality of life. Rarely, a malfunctioning device can cause painful stimulation. The device can be explanted if it is ineffective or paradoxically increases the seizures. Rarely, the device can get infected and needs removal and reinsertion. You should be aware that it is risky to get an MRI done with a VNS device as the heat induced in the bipolar lead by the MRI can cause injury. The technician should use special settings, lower magnetic strength, and other precautions if it becomes necessary to do an MRI on a patient with a VNS device.

Metal detectors, cellular phones, microwave ovens, and theft-protection devices do not impair the functioning of the device. However, the stimulation may cause a tingling feeling in the throat, hoarseness of the voice, cough, or mild breathing problems. The current intensity is increased slowly, usually in increments of 0.25 milliamperes. If your daughter has tolerance issues, the current intensity can be reduced to previous settings.

92. Is deep brain stimulation useful to control epilepsy?

Deep brain stimulation has been in use for other neurological diseases such as **Parkinson's disease** since its approval in 1997. The use of deep brain stimulation in epilepsy is still in experimental stages. The device can be more or less compared to a VNS device. It has a lead that goes deep in the brain, a pulse generator, and a cable that connects the lead to the generator. Several studies have shown that stimulation of the **anterior nucleus of thalamus** can stop the propagation of seizures. The thalamus is the important relay center for different body sensations. The thalamus has an important role in the spread of seizures. Focal seizures leading to a general convulsion abnormally activate the thalamic reticular structures, which are essential to the development and diffuse spread of the general discharge. Other

deep brain stimulation

A treatment where a probe or electrode is implanted and used to stimulate a clearly defined, abnormally discharging brain region to block the abnormal activity.

Parkinson's disease

A degenerative disorder of the central nervous system characterized by tremor or impaired muscle coordination.

anterior nucleus of thalamus

Thalamus is an important structure in the brain through which all sensory impulses pass to the cortex. Thalamus has different nuclei. Anterior nucleus is one of the nuclei of the thalamus.

nuclei of the thalamus have been the target of stimulation as well. What regions should be stimulated at what frequencies for optimal control of seizures is still not clearly understood. Active research is under way to determine when the seizure starts in the brain and to limit stimulation to only when it is required. The stimulation parameters are poorly understood. We do not know much about the seizure types most responsive to thalamic stimulation. More studies are required to resolve some unanswered queries.

93. What is hemispherectomy?

Hemispherectomy is one of the epilepsy surgeries done for medically refractory seizures coming from one side of the brain (hemi = half; sphere = ball; ectomy = removal). Pathology is diffuse in the incriminated hemisphere, and seizures come diffusely from one side of the brain. Children undergoing hemispherectomy undergo video EEG to confirm the source of seizures. A Wada test is done to assess the language and memory locations of the brain. The epileptic tissue is considered the diseased or nonfunctional part of the brain. Children with involvement of one side of the brain as a result of progressive disorders such as Rasmussen's encephalitis and Sturge-Weber syndrome can be helped with hemispherectomy. Those with other nonprogressive disorders such as strokes affecting more than two-thirds of one side of the brain or destructed areas of the brain after head trauma can be good surgical candidates. This procedure is done only for extreme cases. The child's brain is more plastic than an adult's, allowing the remaining nerve cells to take over the function of the disabled brain. The surgical outcome is better when surgery is performed earlier. About 60% of children become seizure free after hemispherectomy.

Indications for hemispherectomy include:

- Rasmussen's encephalitis
- Traumatic brain injury
- Congenital large strokes either in utero or infancy
- Migrational disorders of the brain such as hemimegalencephaly
- Sturge-Weber syndrome

Anatomical hemispherectomy is one of the most invasive surgeries done to help seizures. This involves removal of frontal, parietal, temporal, and occipital regions of the brain. Only deep structures are left behind.

Functional hemispherectomy is a modified approach in which portions of one hemisphere of the brain that is not functioning normally are removed with advanced neurosurgical techniques. The central portions and temporal lobes are removed, but the frontal and occipital lobes are spared. The band of tissue that connects two parts of the brain, called the corpus callosum, is split. This procedure disconnects the various lobes between the two halves of the brain. This procedure requires cutting open the skull bone. The tough membrane that covers the brain called dura is removed. Nonfunctional tissue is removed and bone and dura are stitched back. **Figure 20** shows the postoperative MRI of the brain after functional hemispherectomy where right (the diseased side) brain tissue was removed and disconnected from the left.

Hemispherotomy is another modified form of hemispherectomy in which **temporal lobectomy** is performed, and white matter tracts of the frontal, parietal, and occipital regions are disconnected.

Epilepsy Surgery

anatomical hemispherectomy

One of the surgical techniques to treat medically intractable epilepsy when one hemisphere is mainly affected and causes seizures that are hard to control with medications.

functional hemispherectomy

A surgical procedure that removes portions of one hemisphere that is not functioning normally and disconnects the communications between the various lobes of the diseased side of the brain and the healthy hemisphere.

hemispherotomy

A surgical procedure for hemispheric disconnection. It is a less invasive surgery compared to hemispherectomy and requires less surgical time.

temporal lobectomy

A procedure to remove part of the brain that is involved with speech, language, memory, and the perception of smell and taste.

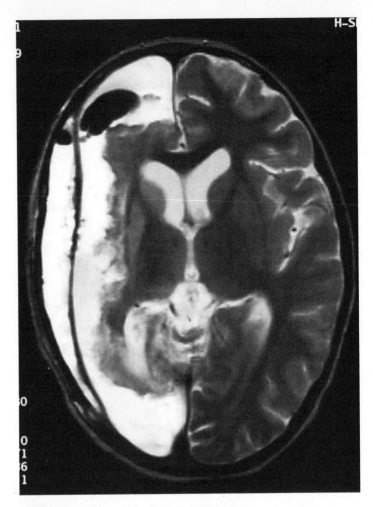

Figure 20
Brain MRI of a child after right hemispherectomy was performed.

94. What are the side effects of hemispherectomy?

There are risks around the operative period as well as late complications of hemispherectomy. Among all epilepsy surgeries, hemispherectomy carries the highest rate of morbidity and mortality, especially in infants less than 6 months of age. The side effects include risk of serious bleeding in the brain, infection, and increased fluid in the brain called hydrocephalus. Hydrocephalus can be an early or a late development. Early hydrocephalus is encountered in children with neuronal migrational disorders. A shunt can be placed in the ventricles to treat hydrocephalus and drain extra fluid away. Superficial hemosiderosis is a late complication of repeated hemorrhage in the ventricles and the sulci seen most commonly with hemispherectomy. Iron builds up in the brain. The iron is in the form of hemosiderin, which is a pigment in blood. Superficial hemosiderosis is not seen with less radical approaches such as hemispherotomy.

Hemispherectomy done at a young age is believed to trigger postoperative transfer of function to the unaffected hemisphere. This is possible perhaps because of the plasticity of the central nervous system.

95. Can patients with tuberous sclerosis be helped with surgery?

Patients with tuberous sclerosis can be helped with surgery. Children with tuberous sclerosis have different seizure types ranging from infantile spasms to complex partial seizures. Tuberous sclerosis is a diffuse disease. However, it is not uncommon to find most of the epiletogenic activity originating from one large tuber. Video EEG and positron emission tomography may help confirm the same tuber responsible for the origin of complex partial seizures. Seizure burden can be reduced significantly by removing large tubers in children with tuberous sclerosis.

More emergent surgery may be warranted, as subependymal giant cell astrocytomas may result in the obstruction of cerebrospinal fluid in the brain. A shunt is used to help drain the excessive fluid from the brain.

Cosmetic surgery or laser therapy is very helpful to tackle skin changes on the face. Partial kidney removal may be needed for tumors of the kidney larger than 3.5–4 cm as these may result in bleeding and kidney failure. Heart surgery is rarely required, because tumors of the heart regress on their own. However, rarely these can obstruct and impair the pumping action of the heart, requiring surgery.

96. What is corpus callosotomy?

Corpus callosotomy interrupts the pathways that transmit information from one hemisphere to the other.

Corpus callosum is the thick band of fibers that connects the two halves of the brain. It has different parts located in the front and the back. A corpus callosotomy cuts the corpus callosal fibers. This surgery interrupts the pathways that transmit information from one hemisphere to the other. Cutting the corpus callosum reduces the severity of seizures. It does not stop seizures from happening, but it stops the spread of the seizure from one hemisphere to the other. Corpus callosotomy requires craniotomy—removing the skull bone flap and the thick covering of the brain called dura. This procedure is done under general anesthesia. Your child may have to miss school for 6–8 weeks.

97. When is corpus callosotomy done?

Drop attacks can be helped with this surgery. Drop attacks can cause severe falls and predispose children to severe head trauma. Corpus callosotomy is also recommended for medically refractory partial seizures that spread to the other hemisphere and cause tonic-clonic seizures. Tonic-clonic seizures carry higher chances of sudden unexplained death during a seizure and predispose patients to significant physical injuries and cognitive dysfunction. Corpus callosotomy is considered a **palliative** but not a curative surgery.

98. Is gamma-knife surgery an option for epilepsy?

Gamma-knife surgery uses a concentrated radiation dose from cobalt-60 sources to damage the abnormal brain tissue. The radiation beams are focused on the targeted area, minimizing injury to the normal structures of the brain. It is one of the least invasive surgeries of the brain, obviating the need for general anesthesia, reducing brain injury and complications of brain surgery, and reducing the hospital stay postoperatively. This technique was originally used to treat brain vascular anomalies such as cavernomas or **arteriovenous malformations**, low-grade gliomas, high-grade **astrocytomas**, and hippocampal sclerosis.

The effectiveness for gamma-knife surgery for epilepsy needs to be proved. There may be temporary amelioration of seizures following radiosurgery. The current efficacy of alternative methods of surgeries limits the role of gamma surgery in patients with epilepsy.

99. What are neuroprostheses?

Neuroprostheses are two devices, one recognizing electrical stimulation and the other delivering drugs to the seizure focus. They are also called hybrid neuroprostheses. They are implanted in the human body. They first monitor the electrical and neurochemical activity from

palliative

Not meant to cure the medical condition but provides significant relief.

gamma-knife surgery

A relatively new form of surgery that uses gamma radiation to destroy the part of the brain that the surgeon has identified as being the cause of epilepsy.

arteriovenous malformation

A tangle of blood vessels in the brain that can bleed and commonly causes seizures.

astrocytoma

A type of brain tumor that is also the most common type of glioma (tumor of the glial cells, the cells that provide support and protection of the nerve cells of the brain). It is most commonly found in the cerebrum (main part of the brain), and it is most common in adults, particularly middle-aged men.

Epilepsy Surgery

the areas of the brain where seizures are originating. They then recognize in real time the onset of seizures and go on to deliver the antiepileptic drug solution directly to that area of the brain. The most common route of administration of the antiepileptics is by mouth. These drugs are then chemically broken down in the body, mainly in the liver. These have to pass through the blood–brain barrier and reach optimal concentrations in the brain. As the drugs are metabolized in the patient's body, they produce significant side effects not only in the brain but in other organ systems, such as liver, blood, bones, and gastrointestinal system, causing toxicity. The idea of neuroprostheses is to deliver the drug when it is required the most, at the onset of seizures, by recognizing the chemical changes and electrical changes just before and during the seizures and then administering the drug. This way the drug bypasses the usual route of metabolism and reaches the brain in the highest concentration, avoiding the side effects of drugs on other organ systems.

100. Where can I go for more information on childhood epilepsy?

It was beyond the scope of this small book to provide answers to all your questions. I have compiled some other good resources, including Web site addresses (see Appendix) that will allow you to get more information on the related topics of your interest.

Resources

Books

Blackburn, L. B. (2005). *Growing up with epilepsy: A practical guide for parents.* New York, NY: Demos Medical Publishing.

The official patient's sourcebook on seizures and epilepsy: A revised and updated directory for the Internet age. Icon Health Publications; an e-book.

Chillemi, S. (2007). *Epilepsy: You're not alone*; Lulu.com, USA.

Devinsky, O. (2008, 3rd edition). *Epilepsy: Patient and family guide.* New York, NY: Demos Medical Publishing.

Freeman, J., Kelly, M. T., & Freeman, J. B. (2000, 2nd edition). *The epilepsy diet treatment: An introduction to the ketogenic diet.* New York, NY: Demos Medical Publishing..

Gay, K., & McGarrahan, S. (2002). *Epilepsy: The ultimate teen guide.* Scarecrow press.

Gordon, M. A. (2003). *Let's talk about epilepsy.* PowerKids Press.

Lechtenberg, R. (2002, 2nd edition). *Epilepsy and the family: A new guide.* Cambridge, MA: Harvard University Press.

Singh, A. (2006). *100 questions & answers about epilepsy.* Sudbury, MA: Jones & Bartlett.

Weaver, D. (2001). *Epilepsy and seizures: Everything you need to know.* Buffalo, NY: Firefly Books (U.S.) Inc.

Other Resources

Acupuncture and Oriental Medical Alliance
Web site: http://www.acuall.org

Alternative Medicine Foundation
Web site: http://www.amfoundation.org

American Academy of Medical Acupuncture
Web site: http://www.medicalacupuncture.org/acu_info/links_of_
interest.html

American Association of Acupuncture and Oriental Medicine
Web site: http://www.aaaomonline.org

American Chiropractic Association
Web site: http://www.amerchiro.org

American Epilepsy Society
638 Prospect Avenue
Hartford, CT 06105
Phone: (860) 586-7505
Web site: http://www.aesnet.org

The American Holistic Health Association
Web site: http://www.ahha.org

The American Holistic Medical Association
Web site: http://www.holisticmedicine.org

American Massage Therapy Association
Web site: http://www.amtamassage.org

American Yoga Association
Web site: http://www.americanyogaassociation.org/

Autism Society of America
Phone: (800) 3AUTISM
Email address: info@autism-society.org

Cyberonics, Inc.
16511 Space Centre Boulevard, Suite 600
Houston, TX 77058-9798
Phone: (888) VNS-STIM (867-7846)
Web site: http://www.cyberonics.com/

Epilepsy Advocate
A variety of camping experiences are available for kids and teens with epilepsy. For a complete list of camps, visit their web site: http://www.epilepsyadvocate.com/resources/camps.aspx

Epilepsy Association of Maryland
For computer programs on the ketogenic diet.
Phone: (410) 828-7700
Web site: http://atkins.com

Epilepsy Foundation of America
4251 Garden City Drive
Landover, MD 20785
Phone: (800) 332-1000
Web sites: http://www.epilepsyfoundation.org; www.efa.org

Epilepsy Parents Information
Web site: http://www.epiweb.org

Epilepsy Therapy Project
Web site: www.epilepsy.com

Finding a Cure for Epilepsy and Seizures (FACES)
724 Second Avenue, LL
New York, NY 10016
Phone: (212) 871-0245
Fax: (212) 871-1823
Web site: http://www.nyufaces.org

HerbMed database
Web site: http://www.herbmed.org

International Chiropractors Association
Web site: http://www.chiropractic.org

Johns Hopkins Epilepsy Center: Ketogenic Diet
Web site: http://www.neuro.jhmi.edu/Epilepsy/keto.html

MEDLINE Plus Health Information: Epilepsy
Web site: http://www.nlm.nih.gov/medlineplus/epilepsy.html

Merck Manual Medical Library Home Edition: Seizure Disorders
Web site: http://www.merck.com/pubs/mmanual_home/sec6/73.html

National Center for Complementary and Alternative Medicine
Web site: http://www.nccam.nih.gov

National Center for Homeopathy
Web site: http://www.homeopathic.org

National Certification Board for Therapeutic Massage and Bodywork
Web site: http://www.ncbtmb.com

The National Institute for Clinical Applications of Behavioral Medicine
Web site: http://www.nicabm.com

Natural Medicines Comprehensive Database
Web site: http://www.naturaldatabase.com

The North American AED Pregnancy Registry
Web site: http://www.aedpregnancyregistry.org

NYSDOH Bureau of Early Intervention
Web site: http://www.nyhealth.gov/community/infants_children/
early_intervention/index.htm

Parents Against Childhood Epilepsy, Inc.
7 East 85th Street, Suite A3
New York, NY 10028
Phone: (212) 665-7223
Fax: (212) 327-3075
Email address: pacenyemail@aol.com

Parent's Connection
Phone: (800) 345-KIDS (1-800-345-5437)

Pfizer Epilepsy Scholarship Award
Phone: (800) AWARD-PF
c/o The Eden Communications Group
515 Valley Street, Suite 200
Maplewood, NJ 07040
Web site: http://www.epilepsy-scholarship.com

Resources for Children With Special Needs, Inc.
116 East, 16th Street, 5th Floor
New York, NY 10003
Phone: (212) 677-4650
Web site: http://www.resourcesnyc.org

Glossary

**2-deoxy-2fluoro-D-glucose
(FDG):** A glucose analogue that is
most commonly used in medical
imaging such as PET. It is taken up
by cells of organs with high glucose
consumption and thereby reflects the
distribution of glucose uptake.

3-Hertz spike and wave: One of the
EEG patterns seen in absence
seizures.

A

Absence seizure: Brief episode of
staring lasting a few seconds.

Acephalgic migraine: Symptoms
such as visual changes, nausea, and
vomiting experienced by a
migraineur; these are not followed by
headaches.

Acquired epileptic aphasia: Regression of language after normal language development.

Activation procedures: Common
procedures done while doing an
EEG. Hyperventilation (deep
breathing) and photic stimulation
(strobe light stimulation) are the

two commonly used activation procedures done during EEG recording.

Acupuncture: A Chinese tradition
in which fine needles are used to
stimulate specific areas along certain
meridians that balance the energy
flow in that area.

Adenoma sebaceum: A skin condition seen in tuberous sclerosis. It
affects face and nose, and can look
like acne.

**Adrenocorticotropic hormone
(ACTH):** A hormone produced by
the master pituitary gland; also used
in the treatment of infantile spasms.

Agnosia: Loss of ability to recognize
objects, people, shapes, smells, or
sounds.

Akinetic seizure: Seizure characterized by brief limping of body and
loss of consciousness.

Allergic reactions: Side effects that
occur because an individual is sensitive to a drug. One example is a rash.

Alopecia: Thinning or loss of hair.

Alpha-fetoprotein: An antigen present in the human fetus and in diseased conditions in the adult.

Alternating hemiplegia of childhood (AHC): A type of migraine that is characterized by vomiting, headache, loss of consciousness, and alternating paralysis/weakness of the body. It is a disease of childhood that sets in before age 18 months.

Ambulatory electroencephalogram: A portable type of EEG that allows the electrical activity of the brain to be recorded over a period of several hours or several days at home.

Amino acid: An organic molecule that forms proteins in living organisms.

Amygdala: Part of the temporal lobe involved in human emotions.

Anatomical hemispherectomy: One of the surgical techniques to treat medically intractable epilepsy when one hemisphere is mainly affected and causes seizures that are hard to control with medications.

Angiomyolipoma: A tumor of fat and muscle tissue that is usually found in the kidney. These are common in patients with tuberous sclerosis, and are considered benign tumors but may bleed, requiring removal of kidneys.

Anoxia: A lack of oxygen.

Anterior nucleus of thalamus: Thalamus is an important structure in the brain through which all sensory impulses pass to the cortex. Thalamus has different nuclei. Anterior nucleus is one of the nuclei of the thalamus.

Antibiotics: Drugs that fight infections.

Antidepressants: A group of drugs used to relieve symptoms of depression.

Antiepileptics: Medications used to prevent the spread of seizures in patients with epilepsy.

Antiviral agents: Drugs used in the treatment of infections caused by various diseases.

Anxiety: Excessive, ongoing worry and tension.

Aphasia: Language disorder resulting from damage to portions of the brain that are responsible for language.

Apnea: Cessation of breathing.

Apoptosis: Programmed cell death.

Arteriovenous malformation: A tangle of blood vessels in the brain that can bleed and commonly causes seizures.

Ashkenazi Jews: Jews descended from the medieval Jewish communities of the Rhineland.

Asperger's syndrome (AS): One of the developmental disorders of childhood. Children suffering from this neurological condition have difficulty interacting with others. Children may experience communication problems as they grow older and exhibit strange repetitive behaviors, unusual rituals, or limited range of interests.

Astatic seizures: Partial or complete loss of muscle tone causing inability to stand, usually with clear consciousness.

Astrocytoma: A type of brain tumor that is also the most common type of glioma (tumor of the glial cells, the cells that provide support and protection of the nerve cells of the brain). It is most commonly found in the cerebrum (main part of the brain), and it is most common in adults, particularly middle-aged men.

Asystole: No electrical activity of the heart; the heart stops pumping.

Atonic seizure: Generalized seizure causing sudden loss of muscle tone resulting in falls to the ground.

Attention deficit/hyperactivity disorder (ADHD): Neurobehavioral disorder characterized by the symptoms of hyperactivity, impulsivity and attentional deficits.

Atypical absences: A seizure type characterized by staring spells that may be associated with eye blinking, strange hand movements, or lip smacking and can be confused with complex partial seizures.

Aura: Warning before a seizure that the patients can recall. It is also called simple partial seizure.

Autism: A developmental disorder that impairs communication and social skills.

Autistic epileptiform regression: Global delays in language and social skills in the second year of life after normal development in the first year.

Automatisms: Automatic or purposeless movements—typically occurring during a complex partial seizure—lip smacking, rearranging objects, chewing or swallowing movements, fumbling with clothing, and undressing.

Autonomic neurons: Brain nerve cells that control those functions that are not controlled voluntarily, such as heart rate, contractions of the intestine, or sweat production.

Axon: Part of a neuron that conducts impulses away from the cell body.

B

Basilar migraine: A migraine associated with complicated symptoms such as slurred speech, loss of balance, or brief loss of consciousness.

Benign familial neonatal convulsions (BFNC): Inherited form of epilepsy that manifests in the first week of life. Newborns suffer from tonic-clonic seizures.

Benign myoclonus of sleep in infancy: A benign sleep disorder that is characterized by rhythmic jerks during drowsiness or asleep.

Benign neonatal sleep myoclonus: A self-limiting disorder in neonates. Neonates have myoclonic jerks during sleep. These movements stop on awakening.

Benign occipital epilepsy: One of the benign forms of epilepsy of childhood with partial seizures associated with visual auras.

Benign psychomotor epilepsy: Also called temporal lobe epilepsy. Seizures are associated with motor, sensory, and psychic components.

Benign rolandic epilepsy: A benign epilepsy syndrome, categorized as partial epilepsy; patients have nocturnal focal seizures with very abnormal EEG, normal MRI of the brain, and normal neurological exam.

Benign sleep myoclonus: A distinctive disorder of sleep in infancy characterized by rhythmic myoclonic jerks (sudden muscle contractions) that occur when the child is asleep and stop when the child is awakened. Sleep myoclonus usually disappears after a few weeks and can be confused with epilepsy.

Bone marrow: A tissue in the hollow interior of bones that produces new blood cells.

Bone marrow transplantation (BMT): Transplantation of the blood cell lines found in the bone marrow from person to person or patients' own bone marrow cells after pretreatment.

Brain stem: Lower part of the brain.

Brain stimulants: Group of drugs that stimulate brain and produce wakefulness and arousal. Examples are amphetamines, methylphenidate, ephedrine, and cocaine.

Brain tumor: Abnormal proliferation of brain cells, neurons, or supporting cells (glia).

Brand name: The name given to a drug by the company that manufactures it.

Bruxism: Teeth grinding at night.

Burr hole: A small opening in the skull made with a surgical drill.

Burst: A sudden appearance of abnormal electrical discharges in the brain lasting milliseconds, seconds, or minutes.

Burst-suppression pattern: An EEG pattern that can be seen in patients who have suffered from severe head trauma or cardiac arrest. Severe multi-organ failures such as liver or kidney problems can produce the same changes in the EEG. This pattern is non-specific and can be seen under influence of sedatives, anesthetics, or after prolonged seizures.

C

Café-au-lait spots: Light brown to dark brown skin lesions with smooth or irregular borders.

Cardiac rhabdomyomas: Tumors of the heart commonly associated with tuberous sclerosis.

Cataplexy: A sudden loss of muscle strength, usually caused by an extreme emotional stimulus.

Cavernoma: One type of malformations of the blood vessels in the brain. It can cause seizures, stroke symptoms, hemorrhages, and headache. It occurs relatively frequently in children.

Cell grafting: A procedure in which

stem cells are delivered or transplanted to repair defective machinery in the cells.

Central nervous system: The portion
of the vertebrate nervous system consisting of the brain and spinal cord.

Cerebellum: Lower part of the brain
that plays a role in coordination and
balance.

Cerebral angiogram: An X-ray of
the arteries and veins in the brain.
For the test, a contrast dye is passed
into the blood vessels through a
catheter.

Cerebral hemispheres: Two parts of
the brain (right and left).

Cerebrospinal fluid: Fluid that runs
in the brain and spinal cord.

Childhood absence epilepsy: Age-
related benign generalized epilepsy
with very brief clusters of absence
seizures; these seizures are also
referred to as petit mal seizures.

Childhood Epilepsy Syndromes:
Age-related syndromes that tend to
have a clinical onset at a certain age,
particular seizure type(s), and unique
EEG pattern. It is important to recognize these syndromes to be able to
understand the best treatment
options and their prognosis.

Clonic seizure: Epileptic seizure
characterized by jerking movements
that involve muscles on both sides of
the body.

Cod liver oil: Oil that comes from
the livers of cod. It is rich in vitamins
A and D.

**Complementary or alternative
therapies:** A group of diverse medical and healthcare systems, practices, and products that are not
presently considered to be part of
conventional medicine.

Complex febrile seizure: Seizure
occurring in relation to high fever,
usually prolonged, and may show
asymmetric involvement of the body
or focal features clinically.

Complex partial seizure: Partial
seizure where the person's awareness
is impaired.

Compliance: Taking medications as
prescribed.

Complicated migraine: Migraine
associated with complex neurological
symptoms such as weakness, loss of
sensations, or visual or speech problems.

**Computerized axial tomography
(CAT) scan:** A brain scan showing
anatomy of the brain using X-rays.

Confusional migraine: A type of
migraine seen in children that causes
a confusional state characterized by
inattention and difficulty with
speech and motor activities.

Consanguineous: Descended from
the same ancestor as another person.

**Continuous spikes and waves dur-
ing slow sleep (CSWS):** Abnormal
EEG findings in an acquired language disorder called Landau-
Kleffner syndrome.

Conversion disorder: A psychological condition in which physical

symptoms arise from the stress at a subconscious level.

Convulsive: Caused by or affected with convulsions (violent involuntary contraction or series of contractions of the muscles).

Convulsive syncope: A brief loss of consciousness (syncope) associated with mild convulsions and stiffening.

Coprolalia: Involuntary utterance of obscene and inappropriate words.

Corpus callosotomy: Disconnection of corpus callosum (*see* corpus callosum).

Corpus callosum: A band of nerves that integrates the functions of the two halves of the brain.

Cortex: The outer layer of gray matter that covers the surface of the cerebral hemisphere.

Cortical dysplasia: A malformed, disorganized cerebral cortex.

Cryptic: Hidden.

Cyanotic spells: Spells associated with fear, trauma, and emotional stress. A child stops breathing, turns blue, and may have a brief loss of consciousness.

Cyclic vomiting: Considered a kind of migraine disorder seen more commonly in children between 3–7 years of age and characterized by bouts or cycles of severe nausea or vomiting that last for hours or even days.

D

Deep brain stimulation: A treatment where a probe or electrode is implanted and used to stimulate a clearly defined, abnormally discharging brain region to block the abnormal activity.

Depression: Chronic feelings of sadness, despair, and helplessness.

Depth electrode: A specialized electrode made of polyurethane or other material that is inserted into the brain to help locate the seizure onset and has multiple contact points.

Diabetes mellitus: Diabetes caused by a relative or absolute deficiency of insulin (a hormone secreted by the pancreas).

Diazepam (Diastat): A type of drug used to treat seizures and is administered by anus.

Diffusion tensor imaging (DTI): Measures the movement of water in the brain and detects areas where the normal flow of water is disrupted. A disrupted flow of water indicates where there could be an underlying abnormality.

Disintegrative epileptiform disorder: Tends to occur between the ages of 2–10 years in autistic children. Children with this disorder can have clinical seizures or abnormal EEG. Children tend to have behavioral issues such as trouble with attention and concentration, mood swings, or cognitive issues.

Divers Alert Network (DAN): A nonprofit organization that ensures safety during scuba diving and prevents underwater injuries.

Doose syndrome: A rare disorder

with frequent and sudden drop attacks, violent myoclonic jerks, or abrupt loss of muscular tone (e.g., astatic seizures).

Drop attack: A sudden loss of muscle tone resulting in falls and physical injuries. The seizures are brief, generalized, and are associated with both atonic and tonic seizures.

Duputyren's contracture: Scar tissue beneath the skin of the palm of the hand. The fingers or sole of the foot can acquire a fixed position. It is commonly seen in patients with epilepsy, diabetes mellitus, and alcoholism.

Dystonia: Abnormal tone of muscle.

E

Early intervention program (EIP): A statewide program, run by Department of Health, which provides several services to infants and toddlers to promote physical, mental, and social development.

Eating epilepsy: A rare form of reflex epilepsy that is precipitated by eating.

Echolalia: Repetition of spoken words by another person.

Echopraxia: Imitation of the observed movements of another.

Electrical status epilepticus of sleep: An EEG pattern showing significant activation of epilptiform discharges in sleep.

Electrocardiogram (EKG): A recording that shows the electrical activity of the heart over time.

Electrodecremental response: Change in the EEG background during an infantile spasm.

Electroencephalogram (EEG): Graphic representation of brain waves revealing the functional status of the brain.

Electrographic seizure: EEG pattern suggestive of seizures without clinical manifestations. Also called *subclinical seizures.*

Encephalitis: Inflammation of the brain tissue.

Enzyme replacement therapy: A medical treatment that focuses on supplementing an enzyme in patients where the enzyme is partially or completely absent.

Epilepsia partialis continua: Continuous seizure activity originating from one side of the brain. Patients may be completely aware of their surroundings. This condition is commonly seen in patients with brain tumors.

Epilepsy: A neurological condition in which a person has a tendency to have repeated seizures—more than two that are unprovoked.

Epilepsy monitoring unit (EMU): A specialized unit where continuous EEG is done; this test is called video EEG.

Epilepsy Phenome Genome Project (EPGP): A research project that is aimed to study the influence genes on the development of different kinds of epilepsy.

Epileptiform discharge: Abnormal

wave in an EEG in patients with epilepsy that indicates signs of excitation in the brain; also referred to as *epilepsy brain waves*.

Epileptologist: A neurologist who specializes in epilepsy.

Estrogen: A general term for female steroid sex hormones that are secreted by the ovary and are responsible for typical female sexual characteristics.

F

Febrile seizures: Seizures in association with high fever.

Fifth-day fits: These usually start on day 2 or 3 of life in otherwise healthy babies.

Flumazenil: An antidote used in the treatment of overdose of benzodiazepines.

Focal seizure: Seizure coming from one discrete focus or part of the brain.

Forced normalization: A relationship between seizure control and psychotic symptoms that exist in some patients with intractable epilepsies.

Forme fruste: A form of tuberous sclerosis where tubers are found in the brain without involvement of other organs such as skin, heart, eyes, or kidneys.

Frontal lobe: The part of the brain that is involved in movement and some aspects of thought, judgment initiation, and abstract thinking.

Functional hemispherectomy: A surgical procedure that removes portions of one hemisphere that is not functioning normally and disconnects the communications between the various lobes of the diseased side of the brain and the healthy hemisphere.

G

Galvanic skin response: Measurement of the electrical resistance of the skin.

Gamma-aminobutyric acid (GABA): A neurotransmitter that inhibits neuronal firing.

Gamma-knife surgery: A relatively new form of surgery that uses gamma radiation to destroy the part of the brain that the surgeon has identified as being the cause of epilepsy.

Gamma ray: Electromagnetic radiation emitted during radioactive decay that has an extremely short wavelength.

Gelastic seizures: Seizures with brief outbursts of emotions, either laughing or crying without any mirth.

Gene: Hereditary material composed of long strands of four molecules that determine the synthesis of proteins.

Gene therapy: A technique that corrects defective genes responsible for disease development. A "normal" gene replaces an "abnormal" gene causing the disease.

Generalized epilepsy: Epilepsy characterized by different seizure types, such as tonic-clonic, clonic, tonic, absence, or myoclonic seizures. These are typically not preceded by any aura and show diffuse involvement of the brain on the EEG during the seizure.

Generalized epilepsy with febrile seizures plus (GEFS+): An epilepsy syndrome with different seizure types such as tonic-clonic, myoclonic, absence, atonic, or febrile seizure.

Generalized seizure: Abnormal electrical activity occurring simultaneously from both sides of the brain.

Generic drugs: Drugs which are produced and distributed after the trademark manufacturers lose their patent protection.

Genetics: Relating to genes.

Gingko biloba (gingko): One of the oldest living trees whose leaves are used in the form of a concentrated extract in traditional medicine to improve thinking, learning, and memory.

Ginseng: A medicinal plant of China that is considered a tonic to the whole body.

Glutamate: An excitatory neurotransmitter.

Grand mal seizure: A sudden attack or convulsion characterized by generalized muscle spasms and loss of consciousness.

Gray matter: The outer surface of the cerebral hemisphere composed of cell bodies of neurons.

Grid: An array of multiple electrodes that is inserted after opening skull bone. It can cover a wider area of brain compared to strips.

H

Habit reversal therapy (HRT): A behavior therapy used in the treatment of tics.

Hemianopia: Blindness in one half of the visual field of one or both eyes.

Hemispherotomy: A surgical procedure for hemispheric disconnection. It is less invasive surgery compared to hemispherectomy and requires less surgical time.

Hertz: Cycles per second.

Hippocampal atrophy: Shrinkage or volume loss in the hippocampus.

Hippocampus: Part of the temporal lobe of the brain that is involved in memory consolidation.

Hot water epilepsy: One of the rare forms of reflex epilepsy caused by bathing with hot water. This is more common in southern parts of India.

Hydrocephalus: An enlargement of the head caused by an abnormal buildup of cerebrospinal fluid.

Hyperactivity/impulsivity: A state or condition of being excessively active.

Hyperventilation: Rapid, deep breathing.

Hypothalamus: Part of the brain that controls many bodily functions such as temperature, sleep, sexual functions, and food intake.

Hypoxia: The prolonged lack of oxygen to the brain.

Hypsarrhythmia: A distinctive EEG pattern associated with infantile spasms.

I

Ictal: The period during a seizure.

Ictus: A sudden event, such as a seizure, collapse, or faint.

Idiopathic epilepsy: Epilepsy in which the cause of the condition is not known but genetic factors are believed to be involved.

Idiosyncratic reaction: Unpredictable adverse reaction to a drug that is not dependent on the dose or the composition of the drug.

Incontinence: Involuntary urination.

Infantile spasms (IS): Clusters of rapid jerks followed by stiffening or jackknife movements.

Inherited metabolic disorders (IMDs): Inborn errors of metabolism. Several biochemical reactions take place in our body. IMDs include defects in the metabolism of proteins, carbohydrates, and fats and certain genetic defects in the cell machinery.

Internal defibrillator device: Device that delivers small electrical energy to the affected heart. This device terminates the irregular heart beat and reestablishes the normal regular heart rhythm.

International 10-20 system: A system where the head is measured between the two bony landmarks (reference points) and then the electrodes are placed at a certain distance. The gap between the 2 electrodes is 10% or 20% of the total length between the 2 reference points.

Intracarotid sodium amobarbital test: Also called Wada test, used to localize speech and memory function prior to epilepsy surgery.

Intracranial recording: EEG recording from intracranial electrodes (electrode grid/strips placed directly on the cortical surface or implanted depth electrode).

Intractable seizures: Seizures that do not respond to treatment.

Ischemia: The prolonged lack of blood supply to the brain.

J

Jeavons syndrome: Absence seizures and myoclonic movements of the eyelids.

Juvenile absence epilepsy: Primarily absence seizures with onset near puberty; myoclonic and grand mal seizures are also seen.

Juvenile myoclonic epilepsy: A syndrome with onset during teenage years, characterized by absence, tonic-clonic, and myoclonic seizures.

K

Kava kava: An herbal medicine that

comes from a plant native to islands of the South Pacific. It seems to help seizures by increasing inhibition in the brain.

Ketogenic diet: A high-fat diet that is sometimes used to treat severe epilepsy in children.

Koenen tumors: Skin growths seen around toe and finger nails in patients with tuberous sclerosis.

L

Landau-Kleffner syndrome (LKS): A rare childhood syndrome in which the child has seizures and regression of language.

Language: Way of communicating that includes comprehension, expression, naming, reading, and writing.

Laser therapy: A treatment using certain wavelengths of light for various medical disorders.

Lennox-Gastaut syndrome: A severe form of epilepsy that usually begins in early childhood and is characterized by frequent seizures of multiple types causing falls and injuries, mental impairment, and a particular brain wave pattern (a slow spike-and-wave pattern).

Localization-related epilepsy: Focal or partial seizure.

M

M-channels: The slowly opening and closing potassium channels that slow down the firing of neurons and exhibit a net inhibitory effect on the brain.

Magnetic resonance imaging (MRI): A brain scan using a magnetic field showing details of the structure of the brain in a three-dimensional way.

Magnetic source imaging (MSI): Superimposition of MEG data on a magnetic resonance image (MRI).

Magnetoencephalogram (MEG): Noninvasive functional brain mapping that localizes electrical activity of the brain by measuring the associated magnetic fields emanating from the brain.

Masturbation: Sexual self-gratification; manipulation of one's own genitals manually or by other means to achieve orgasm.

MECP2 gene: A gene that is important for the function of nerve cells and important to form connections between the neurons (synapses). Defective copy of this gene is responsible for Rett syndrome.

Medically refractory seizures (MRS): Seizures that are not controlled by medical therapy.

Memory: Mental ability to retain and recall different things such as facts, events, experiences, names, numbers, faces, locations, pictures, or other objects and procedures.

Meninges: Three coverings of the brain.

Meningitis: Inflammation of the meninges.

Mesial temporal sclerosis: Subtle scar seen in the temporal lobes in patients with temporal lobe epilepsy due to neuronal loss.

Glossary

Metallic heart valve: An artificial heart valve made of metal that is used in patients when natural valves of the heart are diseased and are malfunctioning. This may require open-heart surgery.

Migraine with aura (classic migraine): Aura characterized by visual changes, nausea, vomiting, and trouble with light and sounds; followed by throbbing headache, pulsating in nature, lasting 4–72 hours.

Migralepsy: An old term that signifies the common association between epilepsy and migraine. It is used in the clinical context when a seizure occurs within one hour after a typical migraine attack with an aura.

Mitochondria: Cellular energy sources.

Mitochondrial disorders: Group of disorders related to diseases of the mitochondria.

Monotherapy: The use of one drug only in the treatment of any medical illness.

Mood disorder: Disturbance of mood such as major depression, mania, or hypomania.

Motor: Movement.

Motor cortex: Part of the brain that controls voluntary movements.

MRI of the brain with seizure protocol: Specialized MRI of the brain that looks at the temporal lobes in a detailed manner.

Multidrug resistant (MDR) epilepsy: Resistance to several antiepileptics.

Multidrug resistant transporters: These transporters promote the outward flow of drugs away from the site where drugs are needed, and thereby reduce the effectiveness of the drug.

Musicogenic epilepsy: A kind of reflex epilepsy where seizures are precipitated by listening to music.

Mutation: Changes in the genetic material.

Myelin: Layer composed of fat (80%) and protein (20%) that insulates the cylindrical part of the neuron called axon. It helps quick transmission of electrical impulses.

Myelination: Process of formation of myelin around the nerve fibers.

Myoclonic seizures: Generalized seizures with brief jerks of the whole body or a part of the body.

Myoclonic status: Continuous myoclonic jerks lasting more than 30 minutes.

N

Narcolepsy: Excessive daytime sleepiness and disturbed nighttime sleep.

Narcotic medications: These are naturally occurring opioid drugs used to treat pain that are derived from the Asian poppy.

Negative myoclonus: Sudden involuntary relaxation of a muscle, rather than a contraction.

Neonatal sleep myoclonus: This is characterized by myoclonic jerks that occur only during sleep and disappears by 2-3 months. EEG recordings are normal in between and during events.

Neural tube: A precursor of central nervous system.

Neural tube defects: Birth defects of the brain and spinal cord.

Neurocutaneous syndromes: Genetic disorders where there is involvement of the skin along with abnormal growth of tumors in various parts of the body and central nervous system.

Neurofibromatosis: One of the most common neurocutaenous syndromes. There are two types of NF—NF-1 and NF-2. Tumors of the nerve cells are seen in NF-1 along with light brown, coffee-colored patches and freckles and eye tumors of the iris and optic nerves. NF-2 is less common and involves the central nervous system leading to hearing loss, loss of balance, and ringing of the ears.

Neurointerventional radiology: A specialized branch of radiology that helps diagnosing and treating disorders of the blood vessels of the head, spine, and neck.

Neurological condition: Medical condition involving the nervous system.

Neurologist: A physician who specializes in conditions of the nervous system.

Neuron: Building block of the brain made up of a cell body, the axon, and the dendrites.

Neuronal migrational disorder: Any defect in the development or the migration or the laying down of the brain cells called neurons.

Neuropathy: Disease affecting the nerves that carry different kinds of sensations.

Neuroplasticity: Reorganization of brain networks and ability to regenerate to a limited extent.

Neuropsychologist: Physician who specializes in the relationship between the brain and how individuals think and behave.

Neuroradiologist: Specialist who uses imaging devices and substances to study the brain.

Neurosurgeon: Surgeon who carries out surgery for the treatment of conditions of the nervous system.

Neurosurgery: Surgery that is carried out for the treatment of conditions of the nervous system.

Neurotransmitter: Small-molecular-weight compound that conveys messages across a synapse. Some examples of neurotransmitters are acetylcholine, glutamate, gamma-aminobutyric acid, norepinephrine, and serotonin.

Night terrors: Episodes of extreme fear, anxiety, or panic within a few hours after going to sleep.

Nonconvulsive: Lacking convulsions.

Nonepileptic seizure (NES):
Abnormal behavior that can resemble a seizure but is not the result of cortical neurons.

O

Obsessive-compulsive behavior:
An anxiety disorder characterized by recurrent, persistent obsessions or compulsions. Compulsions are repetitive, purposeless behavior that the individual generally recognizes as senseless and from which the individual does not derive pleasure.

Occipital lobe: The part of the brain that plays a part in visual perception.

Ohtahara syndrome: A catastrophic seizure disorder with onset in newborns which has different seizure types, such as tonic, partial, or myoclonic.

Organic acid disorders: Congenital metabolic disorders where specific enzymes are absent resulting in accumulation of organic acids in blood and urine.

Over-the-counter (OTC) drugs: Medications that are sold without a prescription.

P

Pacemaker: A small device that is implanted under the skin of the chest or abdomen to control heart rhythms.

Palliative: Not meant to cure the medical condition but provides significant relief.

Pallid syncope: Often precipitated by trauma, a condition in which the child becomes limp and extremely pale with very brief loss of consciousness.

Panayiotopoulos: A recently described benign form of epilepsy where seizures are characterized by nausea, retching, and vomiting. EEG shows abnormal epilepsy brain waves in the back of the head.

Parenteral hyperalimentation (TPN): The administration of an IV solution to provide complete nutritional support for patients unable to maintain adequate nutritional intake.

Parietal lobe: The part of the brain that is involved in perceiving sensations.

Parkinson's disease: A degenerative disorder of the central nervous system characterized by tremor or impaired muscle coordination.

Paroxysmal: Characterized by a sudden outburst or eruption.

Paroxysmal kinesigenic choreoathetosis (PKC): A rare and easily treatable movement disorder. It is characterized by recurrent, brief involuntary "distorted" movements of the body that are provoked by sudden movements.

Partial epilepsy: Epilepsy originating from a part of the cortex.

Partial seizures: Seizures in which the abnormal electrical activity begins in one part of the brain.

Periodic leg movements: Repetitive leg movements of sleep, almost occurring every 20 to 40 seconds, which can last a few minutes to several hours.

Periungual fibromas: Fibrous growths of the toe and finger nails, as seen in tuberous sclerosis.

Pervasive developmental disorder: Broad term that includes autism, Rett syndrome, Asperger's syndrome, childhood disintegrative disorder, and atypical autism.

P-glycoprotein (Pgp): A transporter protein that regulates the availability and distribution of drugs.

Pharmacoresistance: Situation in which medical conditions are refractory to medical treatment.

Phonophobia: Fear of sounds and noise.

Photic stimulation: Stimulation of the brain by flashing light or alternating patterns of light and dark.

Photophobia: An abnormal or irrational fear of light.

Photosensitive epilepsy: A form of epilepsy in which seizures are triggered by flickering or flashing light at particular frequencies.

Photosensitivity: Situation in which seizures are triggered by lights flashing or flickering at particular frequencies and, sometimes, by certain geometric shapes or patterns.

Pituitary gland: The master gland of the endocrine system. It is located at the base of the brain.

Polypharmacy: Use of more than one medication.

Polytherapy: The use of more than one drug in the treatment of a medical condition.

Positron: A positively charged particle that has the opposite charge as an electron. It reacts with an electron to produce gamma rays.

Positron emission tomography (PET): A brain scan that gives information about the function and the structure of the brain. It is a nuclear medicine test in which tissue function can be imaged. Damaged tissues have reduced metabolic activity; therefore, gamma radiation from these areas is reduced or absent.

Postictal psychosis: A state of psychosis occurring after a seizure. *See* psychosis.

Postictal state: A state immediately after seizure is over.

Posttraumatic epilepsy: Seizures resulting from head trauma.

Prescription drugs: Drugs available only by the order of a licensed physician, physician assistant, or nurse practitioner's prescription.

Primary reading epilepsy: One kind of reflex epilepsy that is precipitated by reading.

Progesterone: A steroid hormone produced in the ovary. It prepares and maintains the uterus for pregnancy.

Progressive myoclonic epilepsy (PME): A neurological condition characterized by myoclonic and grand mal seizures, as well as developmental delays. It may have visual, memory, or balance problems.

Proliferation: A rapid increse or growth.

Psychosis: A mental disorder in which delusions and hallucinations are combined.

Pyridoxine: Vitamin B$_6$.

Pyridoxine deficiency: Deficiency of vitamin B$_6$.

R

Rapamycin: An antibiotic that blocks a protein involved in cell division. This drug is also called "*sirolimus.*" It has been used to prevent the rejection of organ or bone marrow transplants by the body.

Rasmussen's encephalitis: An autoimmune disease characterized by intractable seizures as a result of inflammation of the brain. Usually one hemisphere of the brain is spared.

Recreational drugs: Drugs that are just used for fun and not for medical, work, or spiritual purposes. These are called psychoactive substances. A wide range of medications are included in this category such as benzodiazepines, barbiturates, stimulants, and opioids.

Reduced penetrance: The mutated gene effect is modified or reduced and does not always cause disease when present.

Reflex epilepsy: Epilepsy that is triggered by specific stimuli.

Resection: Excision of a portion or all of an organ or other structure.

Restless leg syndrome: Unpleasant sensation in the legs that occurs when retiring to bed. There is almost continuous urge to move legs. Patients find relief by activity such as walking.

Reticular activating system: The part of the brain that plays an important role in arousal and alertness.

Rett syndrome: An inherited disorder exclusively found in girls that is characterized by brief normal development followed by cognitive decline, loss of developmental skills, autistic features, balance problems, and loss of purposeful hand use.

S

Schizandra: Also called *five-taste fruit*, comes from a woody wine found in Northern and Northeastern China. Schizandra is used to improve mental clarity, and to fight depression and stress. It is supposed to enhance concentration and memory.

Secondary generalization: A partial seizure starts from a focus and then spreads within the brain. This process is called secondary generalization.

Seizure: An abnormal clinical behavior as a result of excessive excitation of brain cells.

Seizure alarm: A sensor technology that detects convulsions and triggers an alarm.

Seizure calendar: A calendar maintained by the patient, parent, or a caregiver where patient marks the number of different seizure type(s). A physician can judge the frequency of the seizure.

Seizure diary: A diary maintained by the patient, parent, or a caregiver where the frequency of seizures, duration, and patient behavior during the seizures are recorded.

Seizure dogs: Trained dogs who act as helpers, protectors, and can even sense in advance when a person with epilepsy is going to have a seizure.

Seizure focus: Place where the seizure is originating; if there are multiple sources, they are called seizure foci.

Seizure map: A map of the brain indicating in what part of the brain seizure seems to be originating. It can be very focal, precise, and discrete or can be more diffuse.

Seizure threshold: A person's resistance to seizures that can be inherited. Patients with a low seizure threshold have a higher propensity for seizures.

Sensory: Relating to the senses or sensation.

Shagreen patch: Area of thick leathery skin that are usually found on the lower back or nape of the neck.

Sharp wave: An EEG wave that is broader than the spike (*see* spike). These can last up to 70–200 milliseconds; these seem to arise from some distance away from the seizure focus.

Simple febrile seizure: Seizure occurring in relation to a high fever;

usually a brief grand mal seizure without any focal features.

Simple partial seizure: A partial seizure in which the person remains fully conscious but experiences unusual sensations such as strange tastes or smells, feelings of fear or déjà vu, or involuntary twitching of limbs.

Single photon emission computerized tomography (SPECT): A type of brain scan that gives information about the function and structure of the brain.

Sleep induction: Inducing sleep.

Sleep spindles: A brain activity that happens during sleep. Sleep is divided into 4 stages, 1–4. Sleep spindles are seen during stage 1 and stage 2 sleep.

Sleep talking: Uttering speech while sleep. This is also called *somniloquy.*

Sleep walking: Walking while asleep or in a sleeplike state; also called *somnambulism.*

Slow cortical potentials: Negative or positive deflections on the EEG or changes in the magnetic filed in the magnetoencephalogram that last from 300 milliseconds to seconds.

Slow spike and slow waves: In generalized epilepsies, some waves are recognized by their shape and form, and by the frequency. Slow spike and wave is the irregular burst of spike and slow wave of frequency less than 2.5 hertz. This pattern is seen in Lennox-Gastaut syndrome.

Sodium amobarbital: A barbiturate

drug that is injected into one hemisphere of the brain that can shut down the functions of language, motor, and memory in that hemisphere.

Somatoform disorder: Disorder characterized by a lot of physical complaints by the patient. These complaints sound like medical illnesses but cannot fit into a typical disease pattern.

Spike: Narrow-based waves that have high amplitude. These are recorded from close to the seizure focus and are narrower shaped, lasting 20–70 milliseconds.

St. John's wort: A plant with yellow flowers that is frequently used for depression and anxiety.

Status epilepticus: Seizures continuing for a prolonged time, usually more than 30 minutes, without returning to baseline.

Status migrainosus: A rare, continuous, prolonged, intense, and unremitting migraine attack lasting longer than 72 hours.

Steroids: Natural or synthetic compounds made of lipid and carbon. Common uses in epilepsy include infantile spasms and Rasmussen's encephalitis in children and girls with worsening of seizures around their menstrual time.

Stevens-Johnson syndrome: A potentially deadly skin disease usually resulting from a drug reaction. It can involve skin, eyes, and mouth.

Storage diseases: Neurological disorders affecting various parts of central and peripheral nervous system and other organs where too much of a substance, such as fats or enzymes, builds up in the brain and other organs.

Stroke: Death of brain tissue that usually results from obstruction to the blood flow of the brain.

Sturge-Weber syndrome: A congenital disease present at birth and characterized by a facial birthmark or port-wine stain (reddish brown or pink discoloration of the face). There are malformed blood vessels in the brain that may cause neurological abnormalities, such as progressive mental retardation, epilepsy, and glaucoma in the eye on the affected side.

Subclinical seizures: Seizures that can only be recognized on the EEG, as patient does not exhibit any abnormal clinical behavior.

Subependymal giant cell astrocytoma (SEGA): Approximately 15% of the patients with tuberous sclerosis develop a midline tumor in the frontal areas of the brain that can cause obstruction to the flow of the cerebrospinal fluid.

Subependymal nodules: Nodules that are composed of calcified glia (supporting cells of the brain) and vascular elements that are found in the ventricles.

Subtle seizures: Seen in premature or mature neonates (less than 4 weeks old). Brief blinking, staring, tongue or mouth movements, pedaling, stiffening of the limbs, or just eye deviation can represent subtle seizures.

Synapses: Contact points where the communication between neurons is polarized.

Syndrome: A combination of signs and/or symptoms occurring together indicating a particular disorder.

T

Tandem mass spectroscopy: A tool used for measurement of molecular mass of a sample. This technique is used to understand the composition of proteins, drug metabolism, neonatal screening, and drug testing.

Temporal lobe: The part of the brain that is involved in speech, language, memory, and the perception of smell and taste.

Temporal lobe epilepsy: Epilepsy in which the seizures originate in the temporal lobe of the brain. The seizures are usually complex partial seizures.

Temporal lobectomy: A procedure to remove part of the brain that is involved with speech, language, memory, and the perception of smell and taste.

Testosterone: A potent androgenic hormone produced chiefly by the testes and responsible for the development of male secondary sex characteristics.

Thalamus-cortical network: Important network system in the brain that plays a major role in the spread of seizures and connects the thalamus to the cortex or vice versa.

Tics: Repetitive motor or vocal movements or a combination of both that is difficult to control.

Tomography: The technique of using rotating X-rays to capture an image at a particular depth in the body, bringing those structures into sharp focus while blurring structures at other depths.

Tonic seizures: Generalized seizures, in which a person's body becomes stiff, and he or she may fall backward. The seizure usually lasts less than 1 minute, and recovery is rapid.

Tonic-clonic seizures: Generalized seizures; also called convulsion or grand mal.

Toxic epidermal necrolysis: Severe, life-threatening skin condition that is characterized by blistering and peeling of the top layer of the skin.

Toxicity: Adverse side effects of a drug on a patient.

Tracer: A substance, usually radioactively labeled, that is injected into the patient's body and can be followed to gain information about metabolic processes.

Transporter: Compound that transports different substances within the body and usually across the cell membranes.

Tremor: Involuntary trembling, usually of the hands or head, that can involve the legs, the tongue, or palate.

Tuber: Abnormal, disorganized large neuron cell in the cortex; seen in tuberous sclerosis.

Tuberous sclerosis: A neurological condition associated with seizures, mental retardation, and skin lesions. Multiple organs such as skin, heart, brain, kidneys, and eyes can be involved.

Typical absence: Brief staring and behavioral arrest for 5–10 seconds with 3 Hz spike and wave pattern on the EEG.

U

Urea cycle disorders: Urea cycle is a cycle of biochemical reactions that produces urea from ammonia. Deficiency of enzymes in the urea cycle can cause increased levels of ammonia.

V

Vagal nerve stimulator: A small generator implanted in a person's chest. The generator stimulates the vagus nerve that may prevent the abnormal brain activity that gives rise to a seizure.

Vasovagal attack: A temporary vascular reaction associated with rapid fall in heart rate and blood pressure.

Ventricles: Hollow cavities in the brain filled with cerebrospinal fluid.

Verbal auditory agnosia: Inability to understand spoken language without any hearing problems.

Video EEG: A test involving simultaneous EEG and video recording.

Visual pathways: Pathways in the brain controlling vision or ability to see.

W

Wada: A frequently performed presurgical test before epilepsy surgery. It is also called a language-memory test. It tells your physician what parts of the brain are important for language and checks the memory of the two hemispheres.

West syndrome: A syndrome characterized by infantile spasms, mental retardation, and a specific EEG pattern (hypsarrythmia).

White matter: One of the three components of the brain. It is composed of long processes of the neurons covered by myelin that gives it a white color.

Index

Index